# DO YOU WONDER "WHY ME ?"

## Repeated Patterns of Health Issues Relationship Conflicts Financial Instabilities



**NITIKA JAIN CHOUDHARY**

More than 21 years of Experience as a Clinical Psychologist

BEEJA
HOUSE



**ISBN:** 978-81-19682-27-0 (Paperback)

**Published by:** Beeja House

**Printed By:** Repro India Pvt. Ltd.

First Printing Edition 2024

**Author Email:** divineschooloflight@gmail.com

**Website:** www.divineschooloflight.com

# *Preface*

My sole purpose in writing this book is to bring awareness by educating you on the primary root cause of your health problems, financial instabilities and relationship issues. This book is structured in order to provide you answers to all your questions like "Why me?" It will explain to you how your mind continues to create chaos in your life and you end up wondering, "Why does this happen to me only?", "Why am I suffering so much?"

Through the medium of my case studies, this book will help you to understand that you cannot fool your mind. Consciously, you keep condoling yourself that everything in your life is fine and you are leading a fulfilling life but on the other hand you suffer with repeated patterns of misunderstandings with people around you, financial constraints, severe body pains, hair loss, weight issues, dental or various other health issues. Medicines or meditations only give you temporary relief and you find yourself stuck in recurring problems in your health, finances as well as relationship conflicts. This book will provide you answers to how your issues in health, relationships and finances are interconnected.

As you read every chapter, you will be able to understand that your physical body mirrors your subconscious thoughts which are real reasons for your recurring health problems. It is a myth that hair problems, diabetes, weight issues and many chronic diseases are hereditary.You will recognise that the source of your aches, swelling, breathlessness or chronic diseases is not in your present or the result of your current environment, rather it is your suppressed emotions and negative beliefs formed during your childhood or some past traumatic experiences. The root cause of your anxiety, nervousness, loneliness or feelings of not being good enough are all stored in the form of physical cellular memories as a result of some traumatic past event.. As you will read the case studies, you will be shocked to learn how cathartic moments can be attained in just one therapy session, releasing you from your persistent health struggles, relationship conflicts and financial losses.

This book will not only give answers to all your quests but also provide you with various methods to heal yourself and break the loop of the repeated patterns of struggles in your life. It will teach you that the power lies within you; it is you who has to decide whether you want to be the victim of the circumstance or take full charge of yourself. It will provide you with easy solutions to deal with your health issues and bring a lot of clarity to your way of living. This book will serve as a guide to improve your relationships and financial issues. It will help you to align your mind, body, and soul.

Moreover, the most intriguing part of this book is the past life case studies that are mentioned in dialogue form. If you like to read fiction and adventure novels, then you will find this section of the book most captivating and interesting.

# *Introduction*

**Do you ever wonder why problems seem to pile up in your life, trapping you in every direction; when you feel stuck in one area of your life, then all the other areas also feel stuck.**

When your life seems to be going fine, suddenly you start encountering challenges in all parts of your life whether it is your finances, relationship, or health. Have you ever realized that when you face some financial loss that makes you feel confused and helpless, then you begin to experience that same confusion and helplessness in your relationships and your health as well?

Let's understand this in detail. When you encounter financial challenges then you try to find solutions to deal with your financial problems. You change your job or start a new business, but the work stress continues to build in your mind which triggers disputes in your relationships. You try to amend your behaviour and attitudes to improve your relationships. You try to understand other people around you and do the best for them, but all in vain. You finally give up and try to build new relationships but sometimes you notice similar confusions, frustrations, irritation, and helplessness in other relationships as well. Simultaneously, you develop health issues like back pains, body fatigue, heaviness in your shoulders, or weakness in your legs. You begin to seek medical help, but you notice your money getting more stuck in consultations, medications, and blood tests; and the worst part is when the blood test reports are normal reflecting only slightly decreased vitamins or slight hormonal imbalances. Then the doctors have no answer and they are unable to find the primary cause of your problem. However, based on their assumptions, they prescribe you medications, which may give you temporary relief while the real problem still persists. Ultimately, you find yourself trapped in a vicious cycle of feeling stuck in every sphere of your life in terms of finances, relationships as well as health.

When medications fail, then you try to heal yourself by changing your daily routines, and diet, you begin to exercise, and do yoga and meditations. But you wonder, despite all the diet plans, yoga, exercises or meditations, you get only temporary relief. Have you thought, about why?

This happens because no matter how hard you try to release your current stress, your subconscious mind is still stuck in your past. You continue to heal your present situation but the real problems lie in your traumatic past. Your mind is stuck in the old patterns of feeling helpless in your past episodes of financial lack, relationship conflicts, or health issues which continues to trigger the same feeling of helplessness in your present conditions. This is because you have only consciously moved on while your subconscious mind is still trapped in your traumatic past.

During your childhood when you witnessed domestic violence, domination, physical abuse, or felt neglected, lonely, and abandoned, then you kept perceiving and storing that information in your subconscious mind based on your analytical capacity according to that age. To illustrate, when a traumatic event occurs, a strong emotion is felt that becomes associated with that episode. Your conscious mind draws a conclusion and forms a strong belief about that episode. Intense emotions like fear, sadness, anger, guilt or helplessness, etc. felt during that event also get linked with your belief. Then that negative belief and those painful emotions get stored in the recesses of your subconscious mind. In the future, when another similar traumatic event occurs in which the same intense emotions are experienced, then your subconscious mind triggers the memory of that awful past event. Those negative beliefs or conclusions associated with that painful episode resurface in your conscious mind and as a result, those suppressed painful emotions get triggered in your present. A loop between the past and the present memories is created in your brain neuropath due to which you keep experiencing a similar degree of emotional distress in every sphere of your life — your finances, health and relationships, etc. Your mind feels stuck due to the repeated patterns of torment that drain you both physically and emotionally. This cycle of suffering continues until that loop of the repeated patterns in your subconscious mind is broken.

Healing of the subconscious mind can be achieved through logical understanding and self-realization. When the old beliefs are replaced by new and acceptable beliefs, then you are actually liberated from the old repetitive patterns of health issues, financial stress and misunderstandings with your loved ones.

Have you ever noticed, that when a stranger visits, the child hides behind the curtain and then constantly peeps out to look at the stranger?

Although the child is excited to see a new face in the house and wants to come out, but feels scared to be revealed. When the stranger happens to see this child who is trying to hide, he tries to make the child comfortable and says, "Hello, I can see you, don't feel scared of me, come out. You can trust me." Then the child develops trust and starts showing up.

The therapist's job is similar to this. When the client comes to the therapist with physical symptoms or emotional issues, the therapist assists the adult client in acknowledging and accepting that inner child who is stuck in the memory and this is how the deep healing and integration process occurs. When the inner child is healed, the adult is liberated from the past memories of traumatic events that were preventing them from living their life to the fullest.

For instance, there was a 28-year-old client named Myra, who complained that she had everything good in her life — happy family, friends and luxury, but she felt that there was a repeated pattern of feeling loneliness and sadness. She kept on attracting misunderstandings and conflicts with people around her. She specifically mentioned, "*I keep doing good to people, but they don't do good to me. I keep loving and sacrificing for my loved ones, but they take me for granted. I feel they don't understand my feelings. I mean, I know they care for me, but I wonder why a part of me feels unloved, lonely and unwanted?*"

During the therapy session, Myra regressed to her age of 3 to the moment when her mother was four months pregnant with the second child. Myra felt, "Why suddenly my mother stopped picking me up into her arms?" The 3-year-old Myra was unaware of the fact that during pregnancy, it is advised to avoid picking up heavy weights. The conscious mind of the child kept on analysing that maybe she had committed some mistake due to which her mother was angry. Hence, she decided to obey her mother always. She tried to do her best to impress her mother, but her mother failed to understand the child's emotions. Myra kept on feeling unloved, lonely and sad, and gradually she started believing that *I am the only one who loves and keeps obeying my mother, but she doesn't love me in the same way.* A belief was formed at this stage.

Further, when the sibling was born, mother took care of him more than Myra, as Myra was 4 years old by that time. Myra observed that the mother loved the sibling exactly in the same way as she expected from her. Myra failed to understand as a child that an infant needs more care than a 4-year-old child. Thus, her feelings of loneliness and sadness kept on growing. Gradually, as she grew up, she believed, *I am the only one who loves and cares for people but they don't love or care for me in the same way. I only keep doing good to others, but good doesn't come back to me in the same way.* Her belief continued to confirm with her friends, in-laws, husband and other relatives, and a loop was created.

These strong emotions of loneliness, sadness and feeling unloved were suppressed by the 3-year-old child and continued to trigger repeatedly later in her life. Therefore, the adult Myra felt she had everything in her life, good family and luxury, but still there was loneliness, sadness and feeling of being unloved within her. Through the therapy session, this inner child of Myra was healed and the adult was released from the suppressed past traumatic memories and stuck emotions. After a few weeks, Myra reported that her feelings of loneliness and grief had completely dissipated and she had begun to live a very happy and fulfilling life.

# Contents


PREFACE I
INTRODUCTION III

CHAPTER 1 13
STUCK LOVE, MONEY AND HEALTH 13
**Do you know that the root cause of your recurring health problems is your painful relationships or financial struggles? 13**

CHAPTER 2 21
HAIR LOSS 21
**"I feel anxious about my future." 21**

CHAPTER 3 27
ANXIETY 27
**"I feel anxious and nervous to talk to strangers." 27**

CHAPTER 4 34
EYES 34
**"No matter how hard I try, things can never change." 34**
HEADACHES AND MIGRAINE: 37
**"I feel stuck, confused and lost."** 37

CHAPTER 5 44
EAR 44
**"I feel unheard." 44**

CHAPTER 6 53
NOSE / NASAL ISSUES 53
**"I feel unimportant." 53**

CHAPTER 7 62
THROAT 62
**"I know there is no point in saying anything." 62**

CHAPTER 8 76
SINUS TACHYCARDIA AND SINUSITIS 76
**"I feel lonely and unrecognised." 76**

CHAPTER 9 79
CHEST ISSUES 79
**"I do good to others but never get the same gesture back." 79**
LUNG PROBLEMS AND DISEASES: 80
**"It is my duty to take care of others."** 80
HEART PROBLEMS: 90
**"I feel people take advantage of my goodness."** 90
BREAST PROBLEMS: 97
**"My family is my priority."** 97

CHAPTER 10 105
ABDOMINAL PAINS AND DISEASES 105
**"I feel stuck and helpless." 105**
STOMACH ISSUES AND INTESTINES: 105
**"I get stuck in why? What? And when?"** 105
LIVER: 121
**"I feel angry over people and the entire authoritative system."** 121
KIDNEY: 127
**"I feel angry over parents and siblings."** 127

CHAPTER 11 132
ANAL PAINS AND DISEASES 132
FISSURES AND PILES: 132
**"I feel stuck in my life."** 132

CHAPTER 12 138
JOINT PAINS, SWELLINGS AND STIFFNESS 138
ARTHRITIS: 139
**"Please don't tell me what to do?"** 139
NECK PAIN: 140
**"I cannot tolerate domination."** 140
SHOULDER PAIN: 145
**"I am overburdened with responsibilities."** 145
HANDS AND ARMS PAIN: 150
**"No matter how hard I try, I will never get what I desire."** 150

FINGER PAINS: 158
**"I need to grip control over every situation."** 158
HIP, THIGHS AND KNEE PAINS: 162
**"I have to defend myself, no one supports me."** 162
SCIATICA: 166
**"I cannot sit idle."** 166
KNEE PROBLEMS: 166
**"I can forgive but I can't forget."** 166
LEG PROBLEMS: 172
**"I am always stuck in 'What if? mindset."** 172
BACK PROBLEMS: 180
**"I need support and movement in my life."** 180

CHAPTER 13 189
GENITALS 189
VAGINA AND UTERUS ISSUES: 189
**"My partner doesn't support me in front of his parents."** 189
PENIS ISSUES: 192
**"I feel disappointed and dissatisfied by my life."** 192
PROSTATE DISEASES: 196
**"I feel rejected by my loved ones."** 196

CHAPTER 14 200
URINARY BLADDER 200
URINARY TRACT INFECTION (UTI): 200
**"Life is a big back to back struggle."** 200
BED WETTING: 201
**"I need attention."** 201

CHAPTER 15 203
DIABETES 203
**"I feel rejected and abandoned by my loved ones." 203**

CHAPTER 16 207
WEIGHT GAIN 207
**"No matter how hard I try, I never lose weight." 207**

CHAPTER 17 214
ALLERGIES 214
SKIN ALLERGIES AND ACNE: 214

**"I feel stuck in my boundaries."** 214
FOOD ALLERGIES: 218
**"I feel irritated by my existence."** 218

CHAPTER 18 220
DREAMS AND NIGHTMARES 220
**"Do you wake up in the night and feel stuck; you can't move or speak?" 220**

CHAPTER 19 226
PHOBIA 226
FEAR OF CLOSED SPACES OR CLAUSTROPHOBIA: 227
**"I feel stuck in my life, I need space."** 227
PHOBIA OF HEIGHT: 229
**"I am scared of losing control."** 229
PHOBIA OF WATER: 232
**"I feel suffocated in my life."** 232

CHAPTER 20 235
SPIRITUAL GUIDANCE AND HEALING 235
**HEALTH, RELATIONSHIPS AND FINANCIAL CONDITIONS 235**
LEARN TO CONTROL EMOTIONS 238
CHAKRAS 239
GUIDANCE 248
MEDITATIONS 248
FORGIVENESS 250

SUMMARY - LONG STORY SHORT 252
AUTHORS BIO 254
ACKNOWLEDGEMENTS 257
QUICK LOOK 258
**Dictionary to most of the health problems and their emotional Causes: 258**

# *Chapter 1*
# STUCK LOVE, MONEY AND HEALTH

***Do you know that the root cause of your recurring health problems is your painful relationships or financial struggles?***

As mentioned in the previous chapter, when you face constant challenges in your relationships or finances, your mind feels stuck in an unending loop of negative thought patterns, which activates staunchly suppressed emotions, resulting in health problems and disease. When you feel a certain emotion in anyone sector of your life, you tend to feel it in every other area of your life. For example, in your present situation, if you are feeling irritated because of financial troubles or job, you may feel that same irritation in your relationships as well as health like an irritated bowel syndrome or constant stomach problems.

The clients who complained of severe body pains and health problems found the root cause of their sufferings in the past traumatic memories formed due to challenges in their relationships or finances. The strong emotions felt during any past traumatic event get suppressed in your subconscious mind and continue to trigger in your present, which causes repeated health issues. Let's understand how.

Nowadays, everyone talks about emotions, but do you actually know what the word 'Emotion' is in a literal sense?

EMOTION – E-MOTION, where 'E' stands for Energy. So, the emotion is actually the energy in motion, which is triggered by your thought processes. When we encounter difficulties in our relationships or finances in the present circumstances then our mind triggers the memories of our traumatic past episodes in which we experienced the same emotional turmoil, as a result, the emotion gets intensified and disrupts our entire energy system termed as Chakras. Since emotion is an energy in motion, it quickly resurfaces, and you begin to feel physical sensations. Consequently, you start feeling *Dis-ease* in your physical body.

Disease in a literal sense means illness of your body. It is the uneasiness in your physical and mental body that is caused by the surfaced emotions triggered by your thoughts and perceptions generally encountered after any devastating arguments, misunderstandings in relationships or sudden financial setbacks.

Your brain has an inbuilt autonomic nervous system, which gets triggered during the emergency situations. These inbuilt autonomic nervous reactions in your mind are Fight and Flight. Thus, when there is an emergency situation then you decide either to deal with the problem and confront the immediate issue, which means you try to Fight the situation, or you try to run away, which is termed as Flight. However, in both cases, your stress levels increase.

It is scientifically proven that when your stress increases in your mind then there are hormonal changes that take place in your physical body. Hormones like adrenaline and cortisol are secreted in greater quantities. Excessive adrenaline can cause anxiety, heart palpitations, heart attacks and weight loss; while excessive cortisol secretion can cause weight gain on face and abdomen, fatty deposits between shoulders blades, muscle weakness, diabetes, hypertension, unwanted hair growth on women's face, chest and back.

During the crisis situation of any kind of scarcity or excessive secretions of hormones or extra blood cells, your brain compensates the imbalance.

It helps you to fight harmful diseases and also helps to prevent organ deterioration. When any dangers in your physical body are perceived by your mind, then your autonomic nervous system takes charge. For instance, when there is an excess of bile juice secretion due to bitterness in your relationships, your internal system produces more cells around your liver to protect it from damage; these extra cells accumulate to build a wall around your liver and result in a fatty liver. This stage is a physiological signal by your body to change your negative thought process and heal your suppressed resentment towards your loved ones. As you will read the chapter on liver, you will understand this in detail.

It is your mind that triggers your thoughts and emotions and stores pleasurable or painful memories. Your mind is very powerful, it can be both creative as well as destructive. It continuously keeps playing your thoughts and memories in the background, thus it is essential to have an optimistic outlook. A positive mindset triggers your brain systems, resulting in faster recovery in your health and also improving your relationships as well as financial conditions.

When you suffer from a ligament tear, the doctor prescribes painkillers or in the case of a fracture, places a plaster around the damaged area and asks you to take rest.

**Have you ever thought about who eventually fixes your broken bone or ligament without surgery, is it the doctor or the plaster? When you get a deep cut on your finger and you apply a band-aid, then who heals the cut? Is it the band-aid?**

It is neither the doctor nor the plaster or the band-aid that repairs the damaged parts in your physical body, it is your own mind that helps you to heal. When you take rest then it is your own body and mind that fixes the bone and heals the ligament. Recovery happens far more quickly when you're happy and takes longer when you're emotionally stressed out.

Have you ever noticed that children recover from health problems faster than adults?

The reason behind this is simple. The number of past traumatic experiences of children are comparatively lesser than those of adults. Your subconscious mind tends to fill you up with more and more new beliefs, thoughts and memories of new experiences with age. You carry more emotional baggage than a child. Therefore, it is observed that the recovery rate in children is much faster than in adults.

**Do you wonder why you suffer from severe body aches, fatigue or physical illness after any relationship disputes or financial problems?**

Whenever you experience relationship conflicts or financial constraints then your thoughts trigger emotions like excessive anger, stress, fear or anxiety that leads to physiological changes. It has been scientifically proven that the microscopic view of the DNA of a happy person shows blood cells freely flowing and they are scattered; while the DNA of an emotionally stressed person shows the blood cells squeeze in, accumulate and get closely packed.

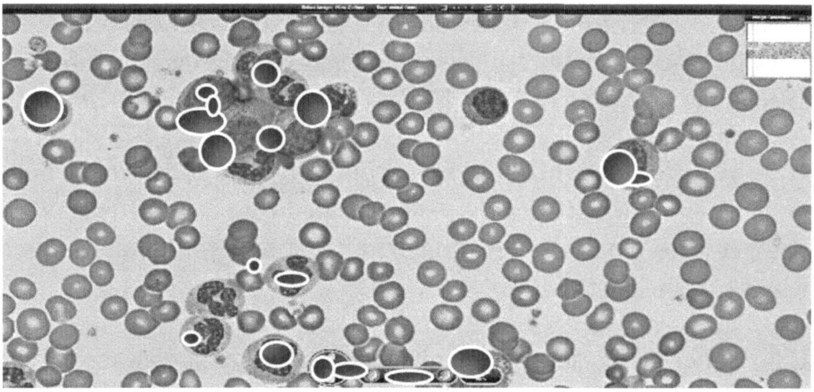

**Microscopic view of the human DNA blood sample.**

This accumulation of blood cells, results in severe body pains, swelling or diseases. The white circle marks and the dark patches in the picture shows the pain, swelling or disease area due to blood cells accumulation. Consequently, you either use pain ointments or oils or hot water bottles to heal the affected part.

Do you know what actually happens by applying these pain oils and ointments? They ease out the accumulated cells which were causing you pain or swelling and as soon as these cells start flowing freely, you feel relief.

In my case studies, I noticed a pattern in the pain and swelling encountered by my clients. The majority of my clients who experienced pain showed a typical pattern of feeling the emotion of guilt, while those who complained of swelling displayed a typical pattern of holding onto hurts and wounds from the past and finding it difficult to let go.

The part of your physical body that experiences pain and swelling is determined by your thought process and beliefs stored in your subconscious mind. For instance, all the clients who came with throat issues agreed that they could not tolerate injustice. Similarly, the majority of the clients who complained of lower back pains confirmed that either their money was stuck or they were facing financial instabilities and most of them had a conscious perception that their loved ones did not support them. You are aware that your backbone supports your entire body. The lower back ache is simply triggered by the negative belief stored in the subconscious mind that *I am not supported.* I would elaborate on this in my book as we address this and various other parts of the physical body in detail with the help of my case studies.

Your physical body only signals and makes you aware of your emotions and beliefs. If they are negative, then they need to be changed, else they would impact your life. Reversal of negative thoughts into positive ones will help you in leading a stress free and healthy lifestyle.

Repeated health issues occur due to the repeated resurfacing of your stored negative emotions and beliefs. These must be completely healed in order to avoid the recurring health problem. For instance, transplantation of the organ is possible, but if you fail to address the deep underlying cause that resulted in the deterioration of your organ, the new organ that you get replaced may be at risk of damage again.

Thus, it is critical to identify and treat the underlying source of the problem and the triggered unhealed emotions. Instead of repressing them heal the primary cause of your problem to lead a healthy life, it's important to clear those negative emotions and beliefs in your mind. By changing your belief system, the cycle of the repeated patterns in your health and relationships can be broken, which in turn can bring an end to your sufferings.

**Case Study**

Naina, a 35 years old client, complained of falling ill repeatedly. She stated in her interview that she had been suffering with a lot of body pains, swelling and stomach issues, ever since she got married at the age of 24. She had started a small business to improve her financial conditions but she always faced financial problems. She wondered why she was always stuck with repeated health issues and financial problems. She said, "Why am I suffering so much? What have I done?" While talking she regressed into the trance state and the Hypnotherapy began; she went back in time to when she was 3 years old and experienced extreme loneliness. She explained that she was the third child and that both of her parents were working, so it was very difficult for them to spend time with her. Her older siblings were also preoccupied with their own lives, such as their schoolwork and friends. She felt neglected, unloved and sad.

Further, she regressed to a memory of when she was 6 years old and she fell ill with acute viral symptoms. She realized that her mother and her siblings started taking care of her. The child observed that her siblings started spending more time with her. Her eldest sister even used to tell her bedtime stories to make her sleep. As a result, the 6 years old inner child of Naina concluded that *When I fall sick then everyone takes care of me.* And this belief was stored in her subconscious mind.

When Naina got married, just after 2 years, when she was 26 years old, she felt that her husband didn't give her time. Her past memories of feeling unloved, loneliness and sadness got triggered, and as a result she started falling sick to seek the attention of her husband. Thankfully her husband was very caring and spent time with her when she was unwell, but since he was in a traveling job, he could not spend much time with her. Consequently, unconsciously Naina started falling sick frequently to gain sympathy from other people. After the astounding session, the 35 years old adult Naina claimed that she had been working and was extremely busy with her work schedules at the age of 28. She was surprised by the shocking revelation of her inner child, who had developed into an attention seeker, triggered as a result of her childhood belief. She consciously acknowledged that she enjoyed being pampered by her loved ones and loved to be the centre of attraction in social gatherings.

**Therapist Conclusion:**

The beautiful therapy session led to an astonishing revelation. 35 years old Naina was falling ill because of her 6 years old inner child, who had formed a belief, *When I fall sick then everyone takes care of me.* The inner child's old beliefs were replaced by the new adult perspectives. Healing process was complete and the adult was liberated from the pattern of falling sick repeatedly. After a few months, Naina emailed to express gratitude because she had completely recovered, was no longer falling ill, and her bodily aches and repeated health issues had also completely cured. She also mentioned that after the session, she noticed her business also started flourishing.

This is an excellent example with an astounding result that will help you understand how your unconscious thoughts and emotions can lead to severe bodily discomfort and illness. Medication can only cure your physical symptoms; it cannot address the underlying emotions that are causing your recurring health issues. The release from the stuck mindset can bring movement in your stuck financial conditions.

As you will read further, you will understand that your body pains are not caused due to exercises or wrong postures because if that was the case then after a few days of rest, your aches and pains should not have persisted. It is your deeply suppressed emotions and limiting beliefs, which are triggered by your past dysfunctional relationships or financial setbacks, that causes recurring, hair loss, weight issues, aches, diseases and various health problems. Your body mirrors your subconscious thoughts; ache in every tissue points at a specific issue in your life. Just by understanding your body pains, you can be aware of the real underlying reason that is causing you repeated struggles in your health, relationships or finances. As you will read further, we shall address the emotional reasons for the discomforts in each body part, in detail which will bring you greater clarity of how your subconscious beliefs affects your relationships, finances and health.

*Chapter 2*
# HAIR LOSS

***"I feel anxious about my future."***

You always find yourself standing at crossroads wondering which way to go; decision making is a task for you as you are always confused with different choices and feel indecisive most of the time.

**Are you always stuck in mental conflicts? Do you wonder that you have been trying very hard but you are never satisfied by your financial conditions or relationships? Do you feel that main cause of your lack could be your bad luck or destiny?**

When you are struggling with money or your relationships then you work very hard to improve your conditions but you are not able to achieve satisfactory outcomes. You feel stuck in an inner conflict; you wonder that you have tried so many different ways to improve your situation, but the lack always persists. This results in hair fall and other scalp related issues. Consciously you are in the impression that you are trying very hard to amend your situation but subconsciously, you may be stuck in certain strong beliefs that are blocking you. Consciously, you may believe that you are a very positive and spiritual person who maintains an extremely positive outlook about life and think positive, but if you are facing challenges in any area of your life then it is because of certain strong beliefs and perceptions formed in your past.

For instance, there was a case of extreme hair fall and increased baldness, who had got the hair transplant done but still he continued facing hair fall issue. He wondered why he could not earn well although he worked so hard and thus, he was always stressed and anxious. Regression therapy was done in which it was revealed that the root cause of his hair loss was his anxiety due to his perceived financial lack. It was discovered through the session that during his childhood, his father used to say, "*Until you work hard, you will never be able to succeed in life.*" Now in the present, the client was in a real estate business; he was very hard working but mostly he worked from home and went into the field when required. He was not working "physically, very hard to earn money." Consciously, he knew that he was working very hard to earn money but subconsciously, he was stuck in the strong past belief that "*Unless he wouldn't work hard, he would never succeed in life.*" He constantly felt unsatisfied and disappointed with himself and thus felt the same discontent and disappointment in his financial conditions as well as in his relationships, especially with his father. Just by replacing the old belief with new and more uplifting beliefs which were acceptable by his logical mind, could help him release from his stuck life situations. In merely one session, he could notice outstanding results in his hair fall. However, he took a session more to increase his low self confidence and self-esteem that was creating obstacles in his work sector. After a few months he testified that his hair fall problems reduced and his financial conditions as well as his relationships had significantly improved. He was very satisfied and felt confident in his approach towards life.

**Do you have fear of the unknown?**

Extreme fear of the unknown is also an underlying cause for your hair related problems like extreme hair loss, baldness, thinning of hair, dandruff or dryness and other scalp related issues.

Whenever you encounter any sudden changes in your circumstances, do you feel frustrated? If you are suffering from hair related problems then change causes you stress and mental discomfort. You only prefer to move on the paths that are known to you; this is because you are subconsciously carrying a fear of the unknown path; this fear makes you resist changes in your life. Try to recall since when are you facing hair problems? You will realize that in the past there would have an event or episodes that caused you extreme fear in your system. You are storing terrible memories of a certain event which triggered the hell out of you. Another cause of your hair problem is the fear that you felt during that moment or during that phase of your life that keeps you stuck with fear of failure in future. Thus, subconsciously you procrastinate and block your own success.

**Case Study**

Justin, 42 years old, was suffering from extreme hair loss. He had tried numerous solutions to stop hair fall but nothing worked. He wondered why? He lost all hope and felt very anxious and helpless. Although, he did not approach me regarding his hair condition, he wished to seek counselling for his anxiety and financial stress. However, his anxiety and mental stress turned out to be a blessing in disguise; via the Regression Therapy session, he found the actual cause of his baldness and was also able to totally heal his anxiety issues. His astounding therapy session will help you to understand how your indecisiveness and overthinking due to your analytical mind can lead to hair problems.

**Therapy Session:**

During the hypnotic session, he regressed to his age of 28 to a phase of his life when he started a new business. He had taken a lot of bank loans which he had to pay back monthly. The therapy commenced in the following way, as he recalled his past memory.

*Therapist: "How did you feel, when you started a new venture?"*

*Client: "I was extremely stressed. I was anxious, what if my business didn't flourish? I was always worried about what would happen, if I would not be able to pay my monthly instalments in time? I didn't enjoy those days of my life. I remember I stopped smiling and suffered so many sleepless nights."*

*Therapist: "Did your hair related problems begin during that time?"*

*Client: "Yes, around that time only. I'm not very sure about the exact time, but yes, during that phase of my life I had extreme dandruff and a lot of hair fall."*

*Therapist: "When you are now overviewing your life, then just tell me did your business flourish?"*

*Client: "Yes."*

*Therapist: "Were you able to pay your monthly instalments in time?*

*Client: "Yes."*

*Therapist: "Today, how do you feel?"*

*Client: "I feel relieved, satisfied and very happy."*

*The therapy session ended with a beautiful self-realization and satisfactory results.*

**Therapy Conclusion:**

It was concluded that the present age 42 years old Justin was at peace as he was a successful businessman and was leading a stress-free life; he was able to clear his loan in time, but the 28 years old Justin was stuck in the past fear of the unknown, and as a result, he was experiencing hair fall and extreme dandruff. After a year Justin shared his pictures, and I was delighted to see remarkable hair growth. He sent me an email expressing his gratitude in which he mentioned that he felt very composed even during the most gruelling times; and his hair fall had also stopped.

**Healing:**

Fear of the unknown, indecisiveness and inner conflicts not only lead to more confusions in your life but also leads to hair related issues as it causes severe anxiety. Overthinking and extreme stress can result in scalp problems. Procrastination and fear of making decisions triggers due to certain past failures in making right choices; sometimes you are not consciously aware of those events but they are stored in your subconscious mind and thus continue to make you feel anxious each time whenever you have to make new decisions. You just need to deal with your fears, don't suppress them under the mask of luck and destiny. The transpersonal therapy sessions can help you to identify and release your extreme fears and anxiety. Regression therapy session is the most effective and fastest way to heal your hair problems as in case of hair related issues it is essential to break the loop of strong beliefs in your mind. If you are facing repeated hair issues then hair transplant can only add new hair, ultimately if you don't change your subconscious negative belief system or subconscious anxiety that is causing you the problem then you will notice that the new transplanted hair will also be lost and your problem will persist. Regression therapies make you aware of the negative entrenched postulates you created in the past as well as the true underlying cause of your hair problems, resulting in better outcomes.

Hair related issues were mostly observed in people who were worried about their finances. Most of the clients claimed that they were not experiencing any financial instabilities in their present, but through the regression therapy it was discovered that they were storing certain childhood memories of financial lack. Thus, they developed subconscious fear and financial insecurities.

In most cases it was observed that clients who suffered with hair problems had issues with their father, either in the present or in their past. They displayed a common pattern of certain strong beliefs or passive anger towards their father that was blocking their financial growth. You may be consciously aware of your issues with your father but if you are not then regression therapy session can help you to understand this better. Deep introspection of your entire situation is a very good way to heal your hair problems. It will not only improve your hair issues but also bring financial growth as well as lead to fulfilling relationships.

Chakras that are imbalanced are crown chakra, third eye chakra and throat chakra. Resolve your inner conflicts and try to focus on the positive. Don't lean back on your past. Bygones should be bygones. Focus on your strengths, appreciate yourself for your accomplishments. Avoid focusing on your weaknesses. Remember what you focus on will increase. This is the law of attraction. If you focus on your shortcomings, then lack will increase. Thus, it's extremely important to focus on your possessions as it will help you to attract more abundance.

Share your thoughts with your loved ones. Expressing your sentiments releases you from suppressed emotions. It eases out the tensions. You feel light and relaxed. Take charge of your thoughts and be mindful of your thoughts and emotions, love yourself. Respect and honour yourself.

While combing your hair, always think positive. Look at your hair while combing and slowly comb your hair, don't rush. Play some light music or sing your favourite song while taking a bath. This is my own experience, and it actually works. Try it!

# Chapter 3
# ANXIETY

***"I feel anxious and nervous to talk to strangers."***

**Do you wonder why you feel nervous when you meet new people?**

Most clients who came with anxiety issues said, "I don't know why I feel nervous, when I meet new people," and a few said, "I don't know why I feel heaviness in my heart?" Some said, "When the time on my watch gets closer to the time when I'm scheduled to meet new people in a social gathering or office meeting, I feel so nervous and experience heart palpitations."

It is not the adult who is feeling this anxiety, nervousness or heart palpitation, rather it is the inner child who is feeling these strong emotions. In fact, the adult (present age) tries to make themself comfortable in front of strangers but because the inner child is stuck feeling scared and nervous, the adult encounters physical symptoms like heart palpitations, sweating or sometimes, unconsciously shaking legs or biting nails, etc.

Your conscious mind is the adult state (present age) that logically attempts to analyse the situation and continue to wonder, why you are experiencing such unexplained emotions? It is the inner child who feels anxious and nervous, not the adult.

As mentioned in the introduction chapter, there are past experiences due to which your conscious mind creates a strong illusionary wall of strength in your subconscious mind to protect your inner child from the outer world as a coping mechanism. This coping mechanism could be a belief or a strong decision taken by you as a child that gives you strength. It helps you to deal with your stress, nervousness and the fear felt by the inner child during that past traumatic event. Under the layer of the new formed postulate, you continue to suppress your unhealed emotions. Suppression of such strong negative emotions is not the solution.

Acceptance is important as it helps you to break the illusionary wall and sets your inner child free from the burdens of hiding your true emotions. Acknowledging your inner child, releases you from all your horrified memories that keep triggering those suppressed unhealed emotions repeatedly. Until the inner child is healed, you continue to feel stuck in the never-ending loop feeling anxious, nervous and scared in every sphere of your life.

**Performance Anxiety**

**Do you wonder why you feel anxious when you have a job interview or have to take any tests?**

People who have taken job interviews have clearly stated that they are the masters in their field and the most capable for the job they applied for, but when they went for their interview, they felt nervous, anxious, restless, and physical symptoms such as current rushing in their blood vessels, weakness in their both legs, sweating, etc. The adult feels physical symptoms and anxiety because the inner child is stuck feeling nervous of being judged. There could be a past memory which is triggered, causing physical and emotional discomforts in the present scenario.

**Do you wonder why a few people keep shaking their legs or playing with their fingers, while talking to you?**

Such people feel restless as they are under immense pressure to achieve goals that are perceived as unrealistic or unreasonable to them. It is not the adult but the inner child that is feeling anxious of being judged. For instance, there was a case of Vikram, 40 years old who complained of feeling very restless and anxious. He mentioned that he used to shake his legs very often, unconsciously. Through the regression therapy it was revealed that that when he was 16 years old, his father pressured him to score well in his exams because it was his father's dream to become an IAS officer, which could not be fulfilled and thus he wanted his son to pursue it.

Further, going deep during the therapy, it was discovered that when he was 6 years old, he was extremely scared of his father as he used to hit him with a stick when he did not wake up early on weekends or when during his school vacations. He was terrified by his father's behaviour and thus he concluded "I have to obey my father else he will hit me." This was the cathartic moment that brought self-realization to Vikram, after acknowledgment and acceptance the wonderful session ended.

**Therapist Conclusion:**

After a striking disclosure, the client consciously highlighted how his father's behaviour had altered after he was 19 years old. He acknowledged that he was unable to pass the UPSC examinations, and his father made peace with him by admitting that perhaps it was fate that neither of them would be able to become an IAS official. Now, when he was 27 years old, he was not scared of his father, at all. After the discussion, it was concluded that at the age of 6 and 16, there were events where he felt traumatized by his father's violent behaviour and remained stuck in those past painful memories. Therefore, whenever the adult Vikram had to go through an interview or apply for a job where he would be judged, then his past memories triggered the same feelings of anxiety, confusion, headache and sweating that he felt during his childhood. After six months from the session, Vikram emailed me a sweet message in which he expressed his gratitude for entirely resolving his tendency of shaking legs.

If you are also experiencing the similar issues then, you just need to acknowledge your inner child, you can seek counselling or Regression therapies to heal yourself.

**Do you wonder why sometimes you suddenly stammer or fumble while talking to a stranger, although you have a good command over your language?**

The root cause is the lack of confidence and fear of failure developed when you were expected to perform well in your childhood. These past emotions of embarrassment and nervousness get stored in your subconscious mind. Consequently, in the present, while talking to the strangers, those past memories sometimes trigger, due to which the anxiety resurfaces, as a result you fumble or stammer. For instance, one of my clients, Samraj, came to me complaining about a stammering problem that occurred while he was making a presentation at his office, otherwise, he never experienced it. There was no reason for him to stammer, as he claimed that he was the CEO and occasionally had to present to his juniors. He felt very confused and wondered why he used to stammer in front of his colleagues? He was wanted to deal with his stammering issue as he felt very embarrassing when his voice fumbled. Thus, a transpersonal regression therapy session was conducted.

**Therapy Session:**

During the therapy session, he went back in time to when he was 3 years old, recalling how he started school at that age and was required to talk in English even though Bengali was his mother tongue. He had trouble communicating with others, which made it difficult for him to make friends in the class. He gradually lost self-confidence as he got older and started to feel inferior. When he was 7 years old, the teacher asked him to read a paragraph from a lesson. Because he was nervous and anxious, he mispronounced the word "lives", and the entire class laughed at him. He felt embarrassed and ashamed, and ever since then, he chose to sit quietly in the corner and refrained from taking part in group activities out of fear of being teased.

However, when he was 14 years old, he formed a group with four friends and served as the class monitor but the painful episodes of age 3 and 7 were parts of his consciousness that remained stuck in the embarrassing past memory. As a result, anytime the adult Samraj was asked to perform in front of an audience, his old feelings of nervousness and anxiety resurfaced, due to which he used to stammer. He felt extremely ashamed and embarrassed.

It was clear that the adult was suffering because his mind was triggering unhealed emotions associated with those past horrified memories. Through the beautiful healing and integration process, the amazing session ended with profound realization and Samraj found the answers to all this "Why's". However, there were two more sessions done with him to completely heal the feelings of inadequacy and build confidence. After two months, Samraj could notice significant improvement in his confidence levels and that he no longer faced the stammering issue, while giving presentations in his office.

**Healing Anxiety:**

Transpersonal Regression Therapies, inner child healing therapy sessions as well as counselling are the faster techniques to heal anxiety issues. However, there are other methods to heal at your level, you can learn about them as you read further.

Positive thinking is very essential to avoid anxiety issues. Focus on your strengths rather than weaknesses. Instead of focusing on what is lacking, emphasize what you have. Your mind needs logic to be happy. You cannot fool your mind. You have to provide valid reasoning to your mind to feel positive else it remains stuck with old postulates.

Focus on your true potentials and strengths to create new beliefs. Remember, *what you believe, you create.* Empower yourself with positive beliefs. If your life seems to be in a rut, then that implies you are bogged down by your belief system. Change your belief system with positive understanding. Focus only on the positive things that you possess, maybe they could be less today, but you have to focus only on the reality. When you focus only on the positive attributes or possessions, it will give your mind logical reasons to feel happy. Remember, you cannot fool your mind!

Writing is an effective way to vent out your unhealed emotions. Journaling or writing your thoughts as diary entries will help you keep a track of your thoughts and emotions. Don't suppress them. Communication is the key to every problem. However, verbal confrontations sometimes may turn out to be hazardous, thus writing is safe a form of expressing your feelings without hurting anyone's sentiments. In this way, your relationships remain intact and your mind feels at peace.

Meditation and yoga aids in releasing stress and helps you in grounding. Intense fear leads to illusions and dissociation. Dissociation causes disoriented minds. You tend to lose track of your reality. Disintegration of thought processes leads to forgetfulness which in turn increases your fears and anxiety. You have to remain integrated with your own true self. Regular meditation and exercises keep you centred and attain peace of mind. You can refer to the meditations given under the "Healing" chapter of this book.

**Self-healing:** Awareness and acknowledgement can aid in faster recovery. Identify your fears, accept them and deal with them. Don't run from your problems, face them courageously. Best way to do so is deep introspection. Try to recall all the positive attributes you possess to fight that fear. Embrace your inner strength and believe in yourself. Build your confidence. You have the courage to accomplish anything you put your mind to.

**Chakras:** Root chakra, sacral chakra and solar plexus chakra are either partially blocked or completely blocked. You can balance your chakras through meditations and positive affirmations. Try to divert your mind to tasks which bring joy to you. Embrace your creativity. Take a more responsible approach to life. Don't let your fears hold you back. Don't dwell into your past. Move on and take action. Liberate yourself from unhealthy habits or lifestyle as you are ready to move beyond. However, you can learn to balance and activate each chakra as well various meditations in detail under the chakra section of this book.

**Affirmations:**

*I believe in myself.*

*I embrace my inner strength.*

*I feel confident.*

*I can deal with every situation.*

*I take all challenges as opportunities.*

**Emotion Management Technique:** You can chant any one word 'helpless', 'fear' or 'anxiety', to feel the physical sensations, then follow the EMT steps mentioned under the "Emotion Management Techniques" section in the "Healing" Chapter of this book.

# Chapter 4
# EYES

**"No *matter how hard* I *try, things can never change.*"**

**Do you wonder that things can never change, no matter how hard you try?**

Then you are one of those who feels that there is no use of complaining as people around you will never change and will never understand you.

If you are suffering from eye ailments, then this implies you don't want to see things around you clearly, you don't want to face reality. You like to stay in your comfort zone. *You don't like change.* You refuse to change your perspective. You don't want to let go of your past. Consciously, you may be feeling that you have forgiven all the people who hurt you, but deep within, you still are carrying the pain in your wounded heart. Let's understand this with the following case study. Following case study will help you to understand that your eyes don't develop redness or start watering due to your present conditions. There is always a reason when any part of your body brings discomfort.

**Case Study**

Ayaan, who was 18 years old at that point, reported that for the past 3 years, during the month of May, he used to develop a significant red clot in his left eye, and also suffered from itching and dryness. He always wondered why in the month of May his eyes developed redness. Doctors said that maybe he was allergic to pollens but he was sure that he was not sensitive to pollens at all. He desired to heal the root cause of his recurring eye problem as he realised that his condition was not just physiological but also psychological. Thus, the Regression therapy was conducted.

A deep hypnotic state ensued and Regression therapy began.

**Therapy Session:**

*During the therapy session he regressed to his age of 6 to the moment when he had got his classmate's Pokemon cards without asking him. When the classmate's mother complained to his mother, she confronted Ayaan. He lied that his classmate gave those cards to him. Then his mother dragged him to the basement and locked him there. There was no light. Ayaan cried out loudly, but his mother didn't open the door. He got scared in the darkness so he closed his eyes and sat down near the door. He felt very hot, he started sweating. He again cried out loudly, but no one came for help. The little child stopped crying after some time. He concluded, "There is no use of crying, no one will come to help me." After a long pause... Ayaan took a deep sigh and said, "My mother opened the door after half an hour or so and I apologized."*

As Ayaan was reviewing the whole episode with an adult perspective, he realized his mistake; He recalled that the incident occurred in the month of May, and that he began to get redness in his eyes in the month of May after that. He suffered from regular headaches and also could not see the black board clearly, so the doctors prescribed him eyeglasses. He confirmed that he had been wearing spectacles since the age of seven. Following Ayaan's deep contemplation and self-realization as an 18 years old adult, the 6 years old dejected Ayaan was healed and the beautiful session came to an end.

**Therapist Conclusion**:

After the awestruck therapy session, it was concluded that when Ayaan's mother closed him in the basement, he got scared and closed his eyes. However, after some time he was relieved, but the 6 years old Ayaan subconsciously remained stuck in that darkness. The emotions of fear, rage towards the mother and helplessness got suppressed in his subconscious mind. He concluded that there was no one for him, so he closed his eyes and decided to stop seeing things clearly. Thus, even though everything was fine after a while, after one year, in the month of May, the suppressed emotions resurfaced.

Any unpleasant emotions that stay trapped in the memory for more than 6 months enters into the DNA and manifests as physical symptoms when the same emotions are triggered again, later in life. Because the tragedy that transpired in May was quite upsetting for the child. May was associated with that painful memory for him. As a result, his suppressed memory resurfaced next year in May, and he developed redness in his eyes, frequent headaches and was unable to see things properly from a distance since then.

You suffer from eye problems because you are stuck in past old beliefs and you don't want to change your perspectives. People around you may feel that you are very stubborn. This happens because you project yourself as a strong headed person, who has a very strong viewpoint. Sometimes you become extremely rigid in your opinions and find difficulty in adjusting to different situations and new people. Consequently, you stop listening to other people. Therefore, it is commonly observed that people who suffer from eye issues, also complain ear problems, knee or joint pains and stiffness in neck, later in their life. You can learn about this in detail as you read further.

As I am writing an accumulative report based on my case studies, I observed that the majority of my clients who had eye difficulties didn't want to be seen by others. They were subconsciously afraid of being seen, therefore they wanted to stay alone and avoided meeting new people. Ironically, all of them had a conscious desire to be recognised and acknowledged. The majority of them were also attention seekers. If you are one of them then you would be experiencing cold or cough very often. As you will read about the cold and nasal issues further in this book, you will understand this more precisely, "Why do you often fall ill with cold and cough?"

## HEADACHES AND MIGRAINE:
## "I feel stuck, confused and lost."

Headache can be pain in any part of the head, while migraine symptoms are characterized by pain on one side of the brain or head. Migraines or headaches occur when your conscious mind gets stuck at some point.

**Do you wonder why in a moment you are physically present, but a part of your consciousness is missing? Do you wonder why a part of your mind is always thinking about something or someone else? Do you easily tune out while someone is talking to you or sharing their life stories with you?**

If you are suffering from migraine attacks or regular headaches, then you struggle with a lot of inner conflicts. You don't want to see the reality. A part of you understands clearly about the facts of life and practicality, but there is a part of you who is stuck in questions like Why? and How?

A clear pattern has been observed, after the therapy sessions of such people, that their half consciousness was missing. All of them were stuck in the past, they kept on thinking, "Why did this happen to me?" or "What will happen now?" or "How is this possible?"

Similarly, until you get answers to all your questions, you feel confused and lost. Consequently, this results in severe headaches or migraine attacks.

Most of my clients who were suffering with headaches or Migraines claimed that they felt confused and disoriented in their daily lives. Do you feel a loss of memory? If yes, you may be subconsciously carrying a fear of loneliness, profound sadness; a sense of being abandoned and a lot of anger deep within you. But you are unable to communicate your true feelings to your loved ones.

**Do you know Anaesthesia is one of the major root causes of migraine attacks?**

It was specifically observed through my case studies that people who suffered from migraine attacks had undergone some sort of surgery before suffering from those attacks.

Actually, anaesthesia is injected before the surgeries and it keeps the patient unconscious for a few hours. Thus, when they regain their consciousness, a part of them remains stuck at the moment when they were in the operation theatre, feeling strong emotions of fear and thinking, "What will happen now?"

Similarly, people who consume alcohol, drugs or are on heavy medication complain of severe headaches or migraine attacks because after consuming them, they become unconscious for a few hours. During an unconscious state, they go very deep in their subconscious mind. When they wake up, a part of their consciousness remains stuck in the past that refuses to come back. As a result, such people are not integrated properly. They often find themselves tuning out of a conversation, they lack focus and feel disoriented.

**Case Study**

Shreya, 38 years old, complained of migraine bouts that were not being relieved by medicines. She had tried allopathy, homoeopathy, and ayurveda and was tired of taking drugs; she became emotionally weak and irritated, feeling stuck in her hunt for the answer to the question, "Why am I suffering?" As a result, she had given up on healing her migraine condition and continuously felt overwhelmed. So, she decided to seek spiritual guidance and heal her emotional state; she approached me for the psychological counselling and discover answers to her questions. Hypnotherapy session was conducted that not only provided answers to her but also healed her migraine completely.

**Therapy Session:**

*Shreya was induced to a deep hypnotic trance state and the therapy began.*

*Therapist: "Since when are you suffering with Migraine?"*

*Client: "For 5 years, I had a slip disc surgery, after that I started getting Migraine attacks."*

*Therapist: "Do you still have back aches also?"*

*Client: "Yes"*

*Therapist: "How do you feel when you get a Migraine attack?"*

*Client: "Oh! It kills me, I feel so helpless, I cannot control it. I feel confused, I feel what will happen now? My mind goes blank and I feel scared. I will not survive."*

*Therapist: "Are you having any headache now?"*

*Client: "No"*

*Therapist: "Go to the last moment when you got this migraine attack. Feel the pain growing."*

*Client started feeling uncomfortable on the chair.*

*Therapist, "What are you feeling?"*

*Client: "My head is spinning"*

*Client started feeling dizzy and had a right side headache.*

*Therapist: "How is it making you feel?"*

*Client: "I am feeling as if everything is going round and round, around me."*

*Therapist: "Where are you?"*

*Client: "I am on the hill."*

*Therapist: "How old are you?"*

*Client: "I am 6 years old."*

*Therapist: "What is happening?"*

*Client: "I am rolling down the hill."*

*Therapist: "Freeze the scene! Now, take all the impressions of the thoughts that are coming to your mind at this moment?"*

*Client: "I feel confused, I am not able to control. I was thinking what will happen now? I feel I will not survive."*

*After a long pause, she said, "I am blank, I can't see anything now."*

*Therapist: "Okay, so now as you are 38 years old and looking at this scene, tell me what happened next?"*

*Client recollected and excitedly said: "Of, yes! Now I remember, I slipped from the hill and rolled down. My mother told me that I fainted as I reached the foothill. They all picked me. I was unconscious for a few hours, then I regained consciousness. I had a severe headache but there was no major injury. I recovered soon."*

*Client started feeling severe back pain at this point during the therapy session, but the session continued.*

*Therapist: "How old is Shreya, who is having this backache?"*

*Client: "32 years old, I had a slip disc surgery."*

*Therapist: "Now, 32 years old Shreya, tell me, when you were being prepared for the slip disc surgery, what were you thinking?"*

*Client: "I was feeling very confused, I was scared as to what would happen? Will I get better or not? I was feeling dizzy and went blank after some time as they gave me anaesthesia."*

*Therapist: "Was the operation successful?"*

*Client: "Yes."*

Inner child 6 years old and 32 years old Shreya were healed.

*Therapist: "Do you feel any dizziness, headache or back pain?"*

*Client: "No, I am feeling fine, now... Thank you!"*

*After the complete integration and beautiful healing process the lovely session ended.*

**Therapist Conclusion:**

Through the insightful therapy session, it was concluded that Shreya was 32 years old when she was preparing for surgery and was puzzled. She was terrified and worried about what would happen, and after a few minutes, she went unconscious due to the effects of anaesthesia. It triggered the past memory of her childhood, when she slipped down the hill. She had been feeling and thinking in the same way while rolling down the hill and had become blank and unconscious in the same way. So, the suppressed emotions related to that dreadful event reappeared. It was the 6 years old inner child who was frozen in that moment and her half consciousness remained stuck in that moment. Therefore, she started getting migraine attacks after her surgery at the age of 32.

It was clear that migraine occurred due to stuck consciousness and the anaesthesia effect but why slip disc? As we have learnt that back aches often occur when you do not feel supported by your loved ones. I inquired after the session from Shreya, did she feel so? She confirmed that she always felt unloved and unsupported since childhood. She added, after her marriage also she never felt the support of her husband and in-laws.

After 2 months, Shreya sent me a written feedback that her migraine had been completely cured and she did not feel dizziness. However, she sometimes felt back pain. You will understand the reason for this under the section of back pain, why Shreya continued to experience back pain.

**Healing Eye Problems, Headaches and Migraine**

Most common emotions observed in people suffering with eye ailments are – disappointment, irritation, extreme fear, stubbornness, rigidity, loneliness and anger. In order to heal the eye problems, you need to release all these negative emotions with proper understanding and awareness. Definitely, you can take Hypnotherapy or any other Regression therapy sessions to tap into the root cause and heal the issue completely. However, at your level, also you can learn to heal your recurring eye problems.

**Self-healing:** "Change the way you look at things, things you look at will change." Sometimes just a slight shift in your perspective can bring profound changes in your life; you will notice that all the bits and pieces will settle in a way that allows you to see things in a new light.

**Chakras:** Third eye chakra and the throat chakra are blocked if you are having eye problems. You have to face reality and your problems.

Do not run from the issues, deal with them.

Affirmation: *"I feel safe to see things clearly."*

Accept change as it comes in life.

Affirmation: *"I feel safe to change."*

Change your belief system. It is a myth that after the age of 40, people develop eye problems and thus face eye issues. Physiologically, only the reading number will increase with age, not the distance number.

**Affirmation:**

*"I create my own reality."*

*"I see everything clearly."*

You often start doubting yourself and sometimes feel guilty of your actions. It's important to accept yourself.

**Affirmations:**

*"I accept myself as I am."*

Tell yourself, it's okay to be seen or noticed.

**Affirmations:**

*"I feel safe when people see me or notice me."*

*"I feel safe when people appreciate me."*

Listen to people, try to understand other people's perspectives.

**Affirmation:**

*"I feel safe to listen."*

*"I feel safe to understand people."*

*"I understand that no one is my enemy."*

Further, the chakra section of this book explains in depth how to activate and balance your chakras.

Practice gratitude and forgiveness. Keep thanking the people who hurt you because they helped you to become so strong in the present. Forgive them with proper understanding and awareness. Acknowledging your strengths as a result of their rude actions is essential. Afterall, they helped you to discover the most authentic version of yourself which was hidden. Release them and release yourself from your wounded past.

# Chapter 5
# EAR

### *"I feel unheard."*

***Do you feel that no one listens to you? Do you wonder that people don't let you complete your statements? Do you believe that there is no point in expressing anything to your loved ones since they will not listen to you? Ironically, you are the one who is not listening to others.***

According to my case studies, individuals who were born in a dominating environment developed a subconscious fear of being dominated by people in their surroundings or of listening to loud voices and so stopped listening, subconsciously. As a result, they developed ear complications later in adulthood. Most of my cases stated that their medical records and tests were normal. So, they were puzzled about why they were experiencing ear difficulties. After the study, it was concluded that it was psychological blockage that led to physical symptoms.

Ear problems that came to me in general were ear pains, blockages and hearing concerns such as not being able to hear well. Some people reported hearing a buzzing sound or whistle, a condition termed as Tinnitus.

**Case Study: Ear Pain**

Sanvi, 41 years old, had been suffering from left earache for the past 3 years and was unable to find the source of the problem medically, therefore she decided to heal her issue through the Regression therapy.

**Therapy Session**:

*Sanvi was induced a deep hypnotic trance state and Hypnotherapy began.*

*Therapist: "Are you having ear pain now?"*

*Client: "It is there, but mild."*

*Therapist: "Breathe into this pain and feel it growing."*

*Therapist: "How is it making you feel?"*

*Client: "I feel… it makes me feel very helpless."*

*Therapist: "Feel this pain and helplessness. Go back in time to the moment, when you felt this pain and this helplessness at the same time."*

*Client started moving her legs restlessly.*

*Therapist: "What is happening?"*

*Client: "I am feeling very uncomfortable and weak in my legs."*

*Therapist: "How old is this Sanvi, who is feeling weak and helpless?"*

*Client: "I am 8 years old."*

*Therapist: "What happened when you were 8 years old?"*

*Client: "I was having a high fever and I was feeling very weak."*

*Client started choking.*

*Therapist: "What is happening?"*

*Client: "I want water, but my mother is not listening."*

*Therapist: "Why is your mother not listening?"*

*Client: "She is talking over the phone."*

*Therapist: "What are you feeling?"*

*Client: "I am feeling helpless, I am choking, but she is not bothered. She was busy chatting…"*

*Therapist: "How did this make you feel?"*

*Client: "Oh! I felt very angry."*

The Client's nose started getting blocked, as she continued…

*Client: "I felt my mother doesn't care for me, as if I don't exist for her."*

*Therapist: "What did you conclude?"*

*Client: "I concluded that no matter what, she never listens to me. So, I decided until she listens to me, I will not listen to her."*

*Therapist: "How did this decision impact your later life?"*

*Client: "I felt that people ignored me when I said something. So I tried to draw their attention towards me. I decided that until they listen to me, I would not listen to them."*

*Therapist: "If they didn't listen to you, how did it make you feel?"*

*Client: "I felt ignored, angry and helpless. Afterall, I can't force anyone. But, yes, if people don't listen to me, then I also don't listen to them."*

*Therapist: "Just go back to that moment, when this ear pain triggered. What happened?"*

*Client: "I had a fight with my husband because he was not listening to me. I was asking for a television remote. I remember, I was not well, so*

*I could not get up, but he kept on working on his laptop and was not bothered at all."*

*Therapist: "How old were you at that time?"*

*Client: "38 years old."*

*After self-realization, the inner children of Sanvi 8 and 38 years old were healed and integrated with current age 41 years old Sanvi.*

*Therapist: "Do you feel any pain in the ears now?"*

*Client: "No."*

*Therapist: "How is your nose, throat and weakness in legs?"*

*Client: "It's fine...now."*

*The lengthy and intense session came to an end with a profound release of unsavoury ideas and emotions.*

**Therapist Conclusion:**

After the deep introspection, it was concluded that when Sanvi was 38 years old, the past memory of her inner child as an 8 year old was triggered, and all the emotions of anger and helplessness surfaced and led to ear pain. The cause of the ear pain was the Symptom Producing Event (SPE). The root cause was the memory of that terrible event as the inner child, who concluded that "No one listens to me, so I will not listen to anyone." During the session, she felt nose blockage, because she felt ignored and the throat discomfort was felt because she felt there is no use of expressing, no one would ever listen to her. You will understand this in detail, as you read further, the chapters on nasal issues and throat problems.

After the session, she consciously told me that everyone told her that she never listened to anyone. She stated that she never let anyone complete their sentences, she always had an urge to explain her point of view first. After a week, she testified that her ear pain was completely healed. She noticed tremendous changes in her attitude and behaviour towards others.

**Case Study: Whistle Sound in the Ear**

Catherine, who was 32 years old, complained of hearing a whistle sound in her right ear for 2 years, so she wanted to take the therapy treatment. Her jaw dropping Regression therapy session was incredible and will leave you awestruck.

**Therapy Session:**

*After listening to the detailed outlining of the presenting issue, Catherine was placed into a deep hypnotic trance state and Hypnotherapy commenced.*

*Therapist: "Are you hearing the whistle right now?"*

*Client: "No, it comes, when I lie down on bed in a silent room."*

*Therapist: "So, just focus on your breath and see yourself lying on the bed."*

*Therapist: "Tell me, how does it feel when you hear that whistle sound?"*

*Client: "I can hear it now, it irritates me; I mean, I feel very angry and helpless, when it doesn't stop. I feel where should I run? I panic when I try to close my ears, but the sound doesn't stop. I don't know, when will it stop now? I feel so anxious."*

*Therapist: "Feel this anxiety and helplessness growing. What is happening?"*

*Client: "Oh...I feel so scared, I can't see anything. I am confused."*

*Therapist: "Look around, where are you?"*

*Client: "I am in an open ground."*

*Therapist: "What is happening, clearly describe?"*

*Client: "I can see people screaming and running. It's a stampede."*

*Therapist: "Where are you watching this from?"*

*Client: "I am also running, I am a Sikh."*

*Therapist: "See in slow motion, what happened?"*

*Client: "I can see people are dying due to gun firing."*

*Therapist: "Did you die there?"*

*Client: "Yes"*

*Therapist: "See your dead body and describe your first thoughts."*

*Client: "It's on the ground, I am a middle-aged man."*

*Therapist: "Just go to the moment a few minutes before you died, get all the impressions, how did you die?"*

*Client: "I see a bullet just crossed very close to my right ear. I can hear a clear whistle sound that crossed me. It didn't touch me. I can see a British policeman standing in front of me, who shot me and then, I died."*

*Therapist: "As you are now dead, just take all the impressions. Why was the British police killing people?"*

*Client started crying with pain and started shivering.*

*Client: "I see, it's Jallianwala Bagh, I went there with my family. Everyone died."*

*Therapist: "That life is now over."*

*Past life was closed and the healing was done.*

*Therapist: "When did that past life trigger in this current life?"*

*Client: "When I was 30 years old."*

*Therapist: "What happened, when you were 30 years old, when you felt so anxious and helpless?"*

*Client: "I saw, "The Legend of Bhagat Singh" movie"*

*Therapist: "What did you feel while watching the movie?"*

*Client: "Oh! I cried a lot."*

*Therapist: "Just try to remember, if you started hearing this whistle sound since then."*

*Client: "Yes."*

*The 30 years old inner child was healed and Integrated with Adult, 32 years old Catherine.*

*Therapist: "Do you hear the whistle sound or any other physical discomfort?"*

*Client: "No."*

*The session ended.*

**Therapist Conclusion:**

It was very clear from the therapy session that when Catherine was 30 years old went to watch the movie *The Legend of Bhagat Singh*, her past life memory got triggered in which she was shot by a British policeman. Firing, gunshot, British soldiers and stampede, all that she had experienced in her traumatic previous lifetime resurfaced and she started feeling anxious and helpless in the same way. The whistle sound that she started hearing after the past life trigger was the memory of the moment, when the bullet in her previous life crossed her right ear, very closely but did not touch her. She panicked and felt helpless. She was frozen in that horrified moment.

After the session, I asked her if she felt that no one listened to her, instead everyone imposed their viewpoints on her. She replied, "Yes," and claimed, "I always feel like people don't listen to me, that they ignore me. I'm quite irritated. I try to convey my perspective, but they refuse to listen to me and instead blame me for not listening to them."

Catherine confirmed that she did not hear the whistle sound after the first therapy session. However, her current life's inner child work was completed in the next session.

**Healing Ear Problems**

If you have ear difficulties, the psychological core cause of the problem, as observed in my case studies, is usually the inner child who stopped listening to others because he or she felt unheard as a child. You may claim to be open to other people's ideas, but you inevitably hold a fear of being imposed by others' points of view, thus you get defensive at the start of the conversation and begin to express your perspectives rather than understanding other people's opinions. Most importantly, feel safe to listen to others point of view. It is fine to listen to another person's perspective and then make your decision in accordance with your intuition. Healthy communication is the key; accept and acknowledge every aspect. In this way you will not stop the flow of the guidance energy that is directed towards. If you are always feeling defensive, then you will not be able to perceive knowledge in its authentic form. Your fear of being suppressed by the other person will always take charge and hinder the situation. You have to be open and receptive.

Your third eye chakra and throat chakra are imbalanced. Third eye chakra is the chakra to see things clearly. Take guidance from gurus, mentors and your karmic teachers. If you will block the guidance coming towards you through them this chakra gets either partially blocked or completely blocked and then you may have problems in your eyes, frequent headaches or nose related issues also. Throat chakra is imbalanced when you are suppressing your emotions. When you feel that there is no point in saying. Thus, it is essential for you to change your mindset. Feel safe to express your point of view as well as listen to others.

You can understand about these chakras and how to balance and activate them in detail in the chakra section of the book.

**Affirmations:**

*"I feel safe to listen."*

*"I understand others viewpoint."*

*"I feel safe to express my emotions."*

*"People understand me."*

# Chapter 6
# NOSE / NASAL ISSUES

## *"I feel unimportant."*

**Do you feel unimportant?**

Then you are one of those who may be catching cold very often or suffering from nasal issues or sinus.

Most common statements of people who suffer from nasal problems, sinus and cold very often are:

*"I am not appreciated."*

*"I feel unrecognized."*

*"People judge me."*

*"I feel ignored or neglected."*

*"I feel irritated but I have no option."*

*"I work so hard, but I never get any credit."*

*"No one understands me."*

Most of them displayed a constant need to prove themselves to others. When there is a *need for recognition*, nose problems occur. However, the emotions truly felt by the individual might vary, depending on the symptoms with which they are experiencing.

**Blocked Nose:** Ego, trying to maintain false high standards. Storing old wounds and past memories of being neglected or feeling unrecognized.

**Running Nose**: Irritation, Helplessness, inner crying and feeling rejected.

**Pain in Nose:** Guilt of helping other people, while they never appreciate or recognize their efforts.

**Bleeding Nose**: Disappointment and anger. Feeling there is no use of working hard, things would never change.

**Case Study**

Loraine, who was 34 years old, complained of a blocked nose and pain. She loved to help people in her community by writing blogs. She used to assist others in her condominium who were experiencing difficulties. She had been suffering from nose issues for the previous 3 years and desired to address the root cause of her condition through the Psychological therapies because she had tried other healing modalities with disappointing outcomes. She mentioned that initially, she felt that she suffered because of cold winds during winters but gradually, she noticed that her nose was blocked during summer season too. She continued to wonder why she always suffered with blocked nose in every season? Doctors said the change of seasons affected her since she had low immunity, but she had a gut feeling that the true cause may be stress, so she approached me to seek stress-relieving therapy. Since, her issue was both physiological as well as emotional, Transpersonal Regression therapy session was conducted. You will be speechless with wide eyes and a fallen jaw as you read her bewildered therapy session, which brought outstanding results.

**Therapy Session:**

*After taking up the presenting issue, Lorraine was induced a deep trance hypnotic state and the amazing therapy session began.*

*Therapist: "What does your nose pain remind you of?"*

*Client: "I have a strong urge to help other people, but they ignore me. I don't understand, why do I need to convince people to take my help, when they simply show that they don't need it?"*

*Therapist: "When people don't want to take your help, then how does that make you feel?"*

*Client: "I feel that they don't know that I can solve their problem, so I keep trying to convince them."*

*Therapist: "When you keep trying to convince them to take your help, but still they don't take your help, how does that make you feel?"*

*Client: "I feel irritated with myself, I feel my mind keeps thinking about them till they understand. I feel my mind gets stuck with them."*

*Observation: Client's nose started getting blocked at this stage.*

*Therapist: "When your mind gets stuck, then how does that make you feel?"*

*Client: "I feel helpless. I feel it's all blocked, I feel stuck."*

*Observation: Client began scratching her nose and started breathing heavily.*

*Therapist: "What is happening in your nose, any physical sensations?"*

*Client: "My nose is getting blocked, and I cannot breathe."*

*Therapist: "How does it make you feel?"*

*Client: "I am feeling very helpless."*

*Therapist: "Keep feeling this helplessness, this blockage. Where are you stuck?"*

*Client started choking and breathing heavily, during the session.*

*Therapist: "What is happening?"*

*Client: "I cannot breathe, something is choking me. I am feeling suffocated."*

*Therapist: "Where are you?"*

*Client: "It is all dark. I feel I am stuck in a small dark cloud."*

*Therapist: "How old are you?"*

*Client: "I am 3 years old."*

*Therapist: "Where are you and what is happening?"*

*Clients choking continued...*

*Client: "It's a small room, it's filled with black smoke. I am feeling suffocated, I cannot breathe, I feel I will die."*

*Therapist: "Did you die?"*

*Client: "No."*

*Therapist: "Watch everything with the bird's eye view and describe what happened?"*

*Client cried: "Oh my gosh, it's a train accident. I can see two trains have collided. People are running out in panic."*

*Therapist: "Where are you?"*

*Client: "I am on the train, it's very dark."*

*Therapist: "Go close to your body and describe."*

*Client cried out loudly: "I am a 3 years old girl. I am crying, but no one is listening to me, no one is even noticing me. I am feeling so scared. My parents left me alone in this darkness. I feel so lost, I am feeling so suffocated. No one is helping me. I can just hear people screaming, I am trying to close my ears but the noise around me is so loud. I feel my body is stuck; I cannot move myself. I feel as if something very heavy is all around me. I cannot move."*

*The Client's past life was closed and the session continued...*

*Therapist: "That life is now over, just view the whole scene from above and tell me, why were you not able to move?"*

*Client: "I can see my father's dead body towards my left and my mother's dead body towards my right. I am stuck between them.*

*Therapist: "Did your parents die in that accident?"*

*Client: "Yes."*

*Therapist: "What happened? How long were you stuck there?"*

*Client: "I can see a few men who rescued me after a few hours."*

*Therapist: "Were you aware that your parents died?"*

*Client: "No, I kept feeling that my parents abandoned me and ran away to save their lives. I spent the rest of my childhood in an orphanage. I felt so lonely. So unloved. I kept quiet in the class and had no friends. Even the teachers didn't notice me."*

*Therapist: "Go forward to see another significant event in that past life."*

*Client: "I began teaching small children, when I was 23 years old. I looked after them. I became the senior coordinator of an NGO and decided to serve those around me. I went to great extent to lend a hand to other people. I promised myself that I would never let anyone feel the way I felt in my childhood, unrecognized, ignored and lonely.*

*Therapist: "When did that past life trigger in your current life?"*

*Client: "I was 13 months old."*

*Client regressed to her age of 13 months, in her current life.*

*Therapist: "Just look around and tell me where are you?"*

*Client: "I am sleeping in my cradle, it is closed from all four sides, so that I don't fall down."*

*Therapist: "What happened, when you were sleeping?"*

*Client: "I heard some loud noise and I woke up."*

*Therapist: "What is happening?"*

*Client: "I am feeling very scared. I am looking for my mother, but she is not there. I am alone. I am trying to get out of the cradle but it's closed from all sides. I am feeling very helpless. I am crying so loudly, but no one is listening to me. No one notices me, ever."*

*Therapist: "How long were you stuck in that moment?"*

*Client: "I slept after some time and my mother came after an hour or so."*

*Therapist: "How did this event impact your later life?"*

*Client: "I developed fear of being alone, I always wanted to be noticed by people around me, so that I am never left alone."*

*Therapist: "How did you make sure that people noticed you?"*

*Client: "I decided to help people. I felt, if I help people then they would tell other people about me, then more and more people would come to me for help and I will never be alone."*

*Therapist: "Now, do you understand, how this decision of the 13 months old child was influencing your life as an adult?"*

*Client: "Yes."*

*The 13 months old inner child of Lorraine was healed and the session was ended.*

**Therapist Conclusion:**

Through the intense therapy session, it was concluded that in her past life Lorraine met with an accident in which she felt stuck, abandoned, lonely and sad. In that lifetime, she heard people screaming due to which, she felt scared and also felt that no one noticed her. While, in her current life, when she was 13 months old, sleeping alone in the cradle, she heard the same kind of loud noise, she woke up and found no one to help her. She felt stuck as the cradle was closed from all four sides, just in the same way as she was stuck in her past life. Therefore, that past life got triggered and all those emotions of feeling lonely, abandonment and fear of loud noise, surfaced. However, later her mother came and things were fine, but the inner child was stuck in that memory, feeling terrified of being alone. She developed fear of loneliness, thus, she decided to help people and desired to always be noticed. But when people didn't take her help, she felt unnoticed, ignored and rejected. Therefore, she was suffering from a stuffy nose and sometimes pain. She also mentioned after the session that since childhood, she had fear of loud noise and was scared of going to crowded places.

After 6 months, Lorraine emailed me stating that she no longer felt distress when people didn't take her help. In fact, she mentioned that she started enjoying her life and spent time with her loved ones. She also testified that her nasal issues also got sorted and she didn't feel any more blockages in her life.

## Healing Cold or Nasal issues

**Do you wonder, you work very hard, but you are never appreciated or someone else takes your credit?**

Now, just pause for a moment and try to recollect. During your childhood or in your teenage, did you feel embarrassed and uncomfortable, when someone complimented you?

One reason for this could be your busy parents, their unrealistic expectations or comparisons. You felt deep within yourself, that no one appreciates your efforts, no matter how hard you try. As a result, you subconsciously develop fear of being judged. You become an introvert and prefer not to be seen or noticed, which affects your low self-esteem and may lead to lack of confidence. But consciously as you grow, you develop a strong desire to prove yourself and a need to be recognised. You are going through a lot of inner conflict and confusions due to which you suffer from nasal issues or frequent cold.

To heal your nasal problems, you must first find peace within yourself and stop proving yourself to the rest of the world. You have to recognize yourself. You must recognise your own accomplishments. When you start to esteem yourself and give yourself importance, you see that the world around you begins to change. Try it!

**Chakra:** When you suffer from nasal issues or frequent cold and cough or sinus, then that means your third eye Chakra and throat Chakra are either partially blocked or completely blocked. As you read the healings for eyes and throat and sinus issues, you can learn to balance these chakras through simple techniques.

However, specifically in learning to heal your nose related problems, you need to see clearly with a positive perspective. For this you can do the following self-healing therapy session.

**Self-Healing Therapy Session:**

Sit down, close your eyes, focus on your breath. Now, feel which of the following statement resonates more to you:

"I feel ignored" or "I feel unimportant" or "I am never appreciated."

Overview your life. Go back in time to the moment, when for the first time ever in this current life, you felt ignored or unimportant or unappreciated. See the whole scene like a spectator. Take a moment and relive that memory. Focus on "What happened exactly, at that time? Why did you feel so? Who made you feel so?"

Now think, as you overview your life, how did that incidence benefit you later in your life? How did it help you to grow into the best version of yourself today?

Thank the situation and the people involved and with this new perspective feel the new emotion growing into you. When you are comfortable you can open your eyes.

**Affirmations:** All affirmations have to be said in present tense and you can say the ones that resonate with you the most.

*"I recognize myself."*

*"I love and accept myself as I am."*

*"I deserve appreciation."*

*"I understand people around me."*

*"People understand me."*

# Chapter 7
# THROAT

***"I know there is no point in saying anything."***

**Do you feel that it is useless to say anything to others as they never understand your point? Are you one of those who can go to any extent to fight for your rights as you cannot tolerate injustice?**

If you frequently suffer from throat difficulties, you are among those who feels that there is no point in explaining anything to other people as they would only understand as per their convenience; you feel that people often misunderstand your intentions and thus it's better to stay quiet. Subconsciously, you are constantly on watch to safeguard your dignity and therefore even though you feel that there is no point in saying anything, you end up arguing. Actually, there is a strong need of justice within you. You cannot tolerate injustice, neither with yourself nor with other people. Just like a lawyer defends his case and never feels shy to put forth his perspectives, you can argue till you prove your point. But with your loved ones all your defences take a toll. You keep suppressing your emotions and need to be understood by them but they fail to understand your emotions. You feel irritated, angry and helpless but never say anything to anyone as you feel there is no point in saying anything as ultimately, it would hurt you only in the end. It is this suppression of your emotions that affects your throat.

Do you resonate with any of the following statements?

*"I cannot tolerate injustice."*

*"I have to fight for my rights."*

*"I feel guilty, I should have said, "blah, blah, blah, but I kept quiet."*

*"I deserve respect."*

*"I think I overreact sometimes."*

*"I sometimes feel I am not good enough."*

*"I feel lack of confidence."*

Most of the people who are unable to express their emotions to others, frequently suffer from throat problems. Most of my clients who complained of throat disorders stated that during their childhood, they could not freely express their emotions of anger, frustration, fear, helplessness, or despair to their parents or teachers. Most of them, who claimed to have witnessed domestic violence or disputes as children, developed a lot of fear and anxiety that affected them later in their life. The clients who were brought up in a dominating environment with controlling parents, relatives or siblings, showed a common pattern of suppressing their emotions as they were scared of getting punishments and thus, they were unable to freely express their true viewpoints as they felt that they would be scolded.

It is mostly noted that such children develop Passive Aggressive Behaviour, which later affects their life as the anger keeps growing with age and when they take charge of their life as adults, then they fight against injustice and for their rights as well as for others.

Further, there were clients who stated that that they were not born in a dominating environment, but their parents and siblings were busy with their own schedules and thus, there was no one to listen to them. It is noted that such children feel confused, lost, lonely and neglected during their childhood. They kept suppressing their emotions and develop feelings of not good enough or inferiority.

However, clients who stated that their parents were intellectuals and expected them to become like them, they were forced by their parents to set big and unreasonable goals, and later pressurized to achieve them. They could never express their true desires. Their efforts were never recognised and always compared with others, and thus they develop performance anxiety, fear of failure and fear of being judged. Such children also kept suppressing their true emotions of helplessness, anger, sadness and suffered later in their life.

In all the above scenarios, it was observed that such children become introvert, they develop lack of self-confidence, low self-esteem and feelings of inferiority, inadequacy, unrecognized and unimportant. They could never communicate their true feelings to the other people, and consequently suffered with throat problems like throat pain, cough, dryness, congestion, thyroid, goitre, cancer, etc.

**Throat Pain:**

Majority of clients who complained of throat pain, showed a pattern of carrying guilt. All of them after the session realized that they were stuck in the past painful memories of resentment and feelings of guilt.

**Throat Dryness:**

Clients who suffered from throat dryness, or dry cough were experiencing irritation, anger and frustration in their present life, mostly due to people around them with whom they are not able to express their true feelings.

**Throat Congestion:**

The other clients who were suffering from congestion showed a consistent pattern of carrying past hurtful memories and a lot of suppressed emotions, mostly anger, revenge and helplessness.

## Throat Cancer:

Clients suffering with throat cancer experienced a common feeling of anxiety and fear of being punished if they did something wrong. Most of them have carried a lot of anger, guilt and helplessness since their childhood.

## Case Study: Throat Pain and Dryness

Karan, who was 26 years old, complained of feeling pain in his throat. He felt as if something was stuck in his throat and had difficulties in swallowing. He suffered a lot of dryness and choking, especially at night which made him feel confused, anxious and helpless. He also complained of acid reflux and stomach upset.

During the counselling session, he mentioned that he had taken all the necessary blood tests, undergone endoscopy and CT scans, but the reports were absolutely normal, and that is why he was confused and anxious. This mental state of confusion and anxiety began to affect his daily routines and his relationships with other people. Therefore, he wished to seek psychological therapies to heal his depression and mood swings. He wanted to find answers to why he was suffering? As his problem was both physiological and emotional, Transpersonal Regression therapy session was conducted immediately. His breathtaking therapy session was extremely deep and intense and as you will read, you will be stunned by the astounding revelation.

## Therapy Session:

*After taking up the presenting issue, Karan was induced a deep trance hypnotic state and the Regression therapy session began.*

*Therapist: "What do you feel in your throat?"*

*Client: "I feel something is stuck."*

*Therapist: "What is stuck?"*

*Client: "I feel there is a lump."*

*Therapist: "Can you describe it?*

*Client: "It is round in shape and black grey in colour, I see blood around it."*

*Therapist: "How is it making you feel, any physical sensations?"*

*Client: "I am feeling pain, it's hurting me."*

*Therapist: "Feel the pain."*

*Client: "Its choking me, I can't breathe."*

*Client: "Oh shit! I can't do this. I can't breathe. I feel like I will die."*

*Therapist: "What is happening?"*

*Client: "I am feeling burning in the stomach."*

*Therapist: "Breathe into this burning."*

*Client's body language changed at this point and he started choking.*

*Therapist: "What is happening?"*

*Client: "I see smoke all around, I am stuck, it's very dark."*

*Therapist: "Where are you?"*

*Client: "I am in the army camp. I am a soldier, I see all camps are burning, we have been attacked by the enemies."*

*Client was breathing heavily.*

*Therapist: "What are you feeling?"*

*Client: "I see blood shed everywhere, I am running here and there to save my people. I am confused, what should I do?"*

*Therapist: "What did you do?"*

*Client: "I am killing the enemies with the gun."*

*Client started feeling restless and anxious and the throat pain started increasing.*

*Therapist: "What is happening? What are you feeling?"*

*Client: "I am feeling guilty and helpless."*

*Therapist: "Why are you feeling guilty and helpless?"*

*Client: "I don't like to kill people, but I have to kill them otherwise they would kill me and my people."*

*Therapist: "Did you die there?"*

*Client: "Yes."*

*Therapist: "How did you die?"*

*Client: "I can see something in the sky, black grey orangish in colour ball, coming towards me"*

*Therapist: "What is it?"*

*Client: "It's like an asteroid, a burning ball or may be its a bomb."*

*Therapist: "What is happening now?"*

*Client: "I'm stuck, everything is over, there is nothing I can do, and I'm going to die now."*

*Therapist: "Did you die at that moment?"*

*Client: "Yes."*

*Therapist: "When in this present life, did this past life get triggered?"*

*Client: "I was 18 years old."*

*Therapist: "What happened, when you were 18 years old?"*

*Client: "I went to a hostel in a different country. I made new friends, but they used to smoke. I used to feel smoking can cause cancer and thus, I tried to avoid smoking. But then I realized that my friends started avoiding me. I felt neglected and lonely. So just to fit in with the group, I started smoking with them. I hid this from my mother because she would never understand, but I had no option. I felt guilty of hiding this from her, but I was helpless. One day, in the middle of the night, I suddenly felt choking and dryness in my throat as if something was stuck. I tried to spit out that stuck thing and saw blood. I got scared, I felt confused. I thought, maybe smoking has caused cancer and now I will die."*

*Therapist: "Did you get the tests done?"*

*Client: "Yes, all reports were normal."*

The 18 years old inner child of Karan was liberated from his trepidation and integrated with the 26 years old Adult. Then the beautiful session ended and Karan was called out of hypnosis.

**Therapist Conclusion:**

It was clear from the Regression therapy session that he started smoking because there was fear of loneliness and feeling of neglect. While smoking, he subconsciously started developing fear of attracting cancer. Moreover, he felt guilty of hiding that from his mother, but felt helpless, as a result when he choked that night and saw blood from his throat and thought that it could be cancer, and now he would die. The memory of the past life of that soldier got triggered in which he used to feel guilty in the same way for killing the soldiers of the other country, but he had no other option otherwise, they would kill him and his people. Thus, he felt the helpless in the same way.

In his current existence, his subconscious mind was frozen in that lifetime. When he saw a round shaped, grey orangish colour bomb heading towards him, and his mind concluded, "Everything is over, I will die now."

When a similar situation occurred in the present life, after seeing the blood, the same thought, "It could be cancer, I'll die now" got activated, resulting in the same emotions of feeling helpless and stuck. After getting all the tests done, the 26 years old Karan was aware that he was absolutely fine and not suffering from cancer, but the 18 years old inner child was feeling stuck in that moment when he saw the blood after choking, due to which the adult was suffering. Just by healing the inner child, the adult was liberated from the trauma and confusions triggered due to the past life. After a few months, Karan confirmed that his throat was completely fine, there was no dryness, choking or pain in the throat.

**Throat diseases like Thyroid or Goitre, etc.:**

Clients who were suffering from thyroid or goitre and other throat diseases, showed a similar pattern of suppressed emotions like extreme fear, feelings of inferiority, unloved, loneliness and sadness. Majority of the clients suffering from thyroid considered themselves as the victims of their environment. They strongly believed that people took advantage of their innocence and they could never say “No” to them. In case of a dominating environment or domestic disputes, there was a common pattern of feeling stuck, rage, sadness and helplessness. They suffered due to their past memories of being tortured or suppressed by the people around them. All of them felt guilty that they never stood up against the injustice towards them or in their environment. Most of them stated that, not only as a child but during their adulthood also they could not express their true feelings to the people around them because they were scared of attracting misunderstanding and conflicts with them and thus, they always suppressed their true emotions and kept quiet.

**Case Study: Thyroid**

46 years old Rama came to me with the issue of hypothyroidism for 10 years and had gained a lot of body weight. She often suffered from cold and cough and body pains.

In her interview, she mentioned that her husband was nice but very controlling. She was very scared of him. She stated that she was the one who was financially supporting the house, paid all the bills and took responsibilities of their children, but her husband who was jobless didn't recognise her efforts at all. Instead kept on fighting with her, she did not have much friends as she often attracted misunderstanding and separations with them. She had issues with her father as well. She felt very helpless, lonely, unloved and sad. She could never express her feelings to anyone because she was convinced that no one would ever understand her pain. She believed that everyone, including her children took her for granted and took advantage of her sentiments as they all were aware that she loved them and so she would never get separated from them. She constantly kept on repeating, "I feel so stuck. I don't know what to do? Why am I suffering? Why did God do this with me, when I have never hurt anyone?"

In such cases, where client is extremely depressed and convinced that there is no cure to their sufferings, Transpersonal Regression therapy is the most effective way to bring deep introspection and self-realization; thus, the Regression therapy session was conducted to seek answers to all her questions which brought astonishing results.

**Therapy Session:**

*Rama was induced a deep trance hypnotic state and the Regression therapy session commenced.*

*Therapist: "Any pain right now?"*

*Client: "No."*

*Therapist: "What hurts you the most?"*

*Client: "I feel that no one understands me."*

*Therapist: "How does it make you feel?"*

*Client: "I feel there is no point in explaining anything, they will not understand."*

*Therapist: "How does that make you feel?"*

*Client: "I feel confused sometimes, there is a part of me that says that I should express my feelings, but at the same time there is another part of me that feels that it's pointless to say anything, it's better to keep quiet."*

*Therapist: "How does that make you feel?"*

*Client: "I feel helpless."*

*Therapist: "Repeat the word 'Helpless'. Feel this helplessness growing in your body."*

*Client: "Helpless, Helpless, Helpless..."*

*Therapist: "Any physical sensations?"*

*Client: "Yes, I am getting pain in my arms, heaviness in the chest, pain in the shoulders and dryness in the throat."*

*Therapist: "Feel the sensations, and choose the strongest one?"*

*Client: "I feel something is stuck in my throat, I cannot swallow."*

*Therapist: "How does it make you feel?"*

*Client: "I feel helpless, I am stuck."*

*Therapist: "Where are you stuck? Look around."*

*Client: "It's a very crowded place."*

*Therapist: "How old are you?"*

*Client: "I am 5 years old."*

*Therapist: "What happened, when you were five years old?"*

*Client: "I am crying, I am feeling confused. I am lost in the crowded fair. I am finding my mother and father."*

*Therapist: "Did you find your mother and father?"*

*Client: "Yes, after some time, my father found me."*

*Therapist: "What happened then?"*

*Client: "When I saw my father, I ran towards him to hug him. I was so happy to see him, but he shouted at me and scolded me for not holding his hand in that crowded place and made me feel guilty."*

*Therapist: "How is the child feeling?"*

*Client: "I am feeling very confused, because I was feeling that my father didn't even let me hug him, he did not even ask me, how I was feeling? He kept on blaming me for being careless and getting lost. I tried to explain myself to him, but he didn't listen to me, he kept on and on and on..."*

*Therapist: "What did the 5 years old child conclude?"*

*Client: "I concluded that there is no point in telling him anything, he will never understand me. It's better to keep quiet, else he would scold me more."*

*Therapist: "Do you feel that later, when you grew up, your father listened to your viewpoints?"*

*Client: "Yes, he is dominating, and I am still scared of him but not that much, now, we share a good bond."*

Rama was able to realise the fundamental reason of her acrimony near the end of the enlightening session. Rama's 5 years old inner child was healed, and the most intense session came to an end.

**Therapist Conclusion:**

The beautiful session concluded with a deep insight and self-realization by the adult that it was the inner child who was stuck in the past memory and believed that there is no use of explaining to others as they would not listen to her. The inner child was healed, and the negative belief cycle was broken. The adult was then liberated from the cycle of attracting misunderstandings and disputes with those around her as a result of a communication gap.

After a few months, Rama testified that her conflicts with her husband reduced because she was able to explain her points of view to him after the therapy session, and he also understood her sentiments. She told me that she had become very social and that she no longer felt lonely or unloved. Although it was very lengthy, it was a very satisfying session. Moreover, lovely feedback from my clients were always inspiring and pushed me to keep on healing selflessly.

**Healing Throat Problems:**

**To heal the throat issues, it is extremely important for you to express your emotions clearly while maintaining a perfect balance and harmony of your relationship with the other person.** You are your best attorney. The power of being your own attorney is in your hands. Don't expect others to stand in for you or defend you from any attacks because you are capable of doing it. Follow the strength that you exhibit, just like an attorney. You can be assured of emerging victorious in all your encounters. But the key to emerge victorious is mutual respect and considering other persons perspectives as well.

Live life possessing the character of being dauntless, such that you can claim for the right treatment for your shortcomings. Just like a good lawyer makes logical justifications and does not shy away from speaking out clearly that he wants to communicate, attain the power of being your own attorney of life.

You ought to be proactive and voice out the challenges you are encountering. But whatever you do, keep in mind to positively introspect *the situations and the point of views of other people*. Have an optimistic outlook. Just like a spectator, come out of the situation and analyse it, in view of both the parties.

As mentioned earlier under the nasal issue chapter, as a result of parental pressures and expectations, during your childhood you develop lack of confidence and feelings of not good enough, which may have made you feel that you were not worthy. Consequently, subconsciously you have concluded, "*I don't deserve.*" To heal the throat issues, such self-limiting beliefs have to be changed. This can be done through positive thinking and affirmations at conscious level. When you do the affirmations, then say positive statements in present tense like:

*"I am worthy."*

*"I feel confident."*

*"I can express freely."*

*"I deserve happiness."*

*"I deserve respect."*

*"I feel safe to speak for myself."*

*"I feel safe to communicate my ideas."*

Remember affirmations work only if they are logical and your mind accepts them, so always say with proper understanding. Overview your life and see the bigger picture. How did a particular person or situation benefit you? How did it help you to grow and evolve and make you a better person?

However, if there is a blockage in the subconscious mind, then affirmations may not work. In that case, Hypnotherapy sessions are required to heal the root cause.

Chakras: If you are suffering from the throat problems often, then your third eye chakra, throat chakra, and your heart chakra are either partially blocked or completely blocked. Third eye chakra is the chakra of understanding and to see things clearly. Generally, the throat problem begins when you are not able to understand the perspective of the other person. Then you hold yourself back and you don't want to communicate clearly. As a result, your third eye chakra as well as your throat chakra become imbalanced. Consequently, you end up having relationship issues with most of the people around you, due to which your heart chakra also gets affected and becomes imbalanced.

This book's chakra section describes in detail how to activate and balance all of your chakras. As you read the chakra section, you will gain a greater understanding of this.

# Chapter 8
# SINUS TACHYCARDIA AND SINUSITIS

***"I feel lonely and unrecognised."***

**Do you feel lonely and unrecognised?**

Majority of the clients who suffered from Sinus, or cold and sneezing, felt lonely and abandoned by their loved ones. They felt that they were never recognised by them. They felt that not only their loved ones but the other people also ignored them. They felt all the emotions that are experienced by people who suffer from Nasal and throat issues. They could never express their true feelings. They were scared of losing people they loved and thus they continued to tolerate their hostile behaviour and never stood up for their rights.

**Case Study**

Presenting Issue: Sinus and sneezing when there was dust, smoke or visited old buildings.

Sunita, who was 53 years old, was suffering from sinus. She also mentioned in her first counselling session that she was allergic to dust and smoke. She used to sneeze when she visited any old tombs or archaeological buildings. She stated that her mother also suffered from this same issue. She had one brother and three sisters, but she was the only one who inherited this issue from the mother. She wanted to know, "Why me only? Why did I inherit sinus from my mother and not any other siblings?" The way all of her above issues got connected and answered to all her questions was very intriguing. The astonishing outcomes of the therapy session are surely going to stun you and bring you awareness about how the complications of our mind effects not only our health but also our beautiful relationships.

**Therapy Session:**

Hypnotherapy session was conducted. During the deep trance state, Sunita regressed to her past life to the moment when she saw herself as a 60 years old lady, who lived in a huge old heritage property in a desert. She had children and grandchildren, but no one cared for her. She felt very lonely and sad. She died at the age of 65 as the house caught fire. No one came to help her. While dying she could see only smoke (she started choking in the session).

In the hypnotic state, she said that she tried to run out of the house due to which she caught fire and died in a lot of pain and feeling helpless on the sand thinking, "Why did this happen to me? What did I do? What was my mistake?" Exactly the same questions that she was curious to know before the therapy session began.

That past life got triggered in her current life when she was 2 years old. I asked her, "What happened when she was 2 years old?" She said that she fell ill with smallpox, so her parents left her with her grandmother as they both were busy with their jobs and did not have time to take care of her. She cried out loudly, "They abandoned me, I felt so lonely. Why did they do this to me, what was my mistake?"

Since in her past life, she died due to fire, thus, the burning felt on her skin and marks formed due to smallpox in her current life when she was 2 years old, triggered that past life. As a result, all the emotions felt in that lifetime also surfaced. She started feeling lonely, sad and helpless as parents left her alone with her grandmother. Since then, she continuously complained of dryness in her eyes and throat, her nose was always blocked, she used to sneeze when there was dust around her. When she was 6 years old, she was diagnosed with sinus. With growing age, sinus continuously kept on increasing and it became worse when she visited old buildings, deserts or saw smoke.

After the session, Sunita consciously told me that she felt unimportant and there was a desire in her to be recognized and appreciated. She told me that when she was 6 years old her parents brought her back home, and since then she used to work very hard to impress her parents. She tried to score good marks, she tried to help her mother in the kitchen, she obeyed them always, but she continued to feel unloved and felt that she was always compared to her younger sister. She mentioned that she had a fear of being left alone, thus, when she joined college, she tried to be socially active and she always tried to be the centre of attraction in the group, so that she could feel important among people.

It was the 2 years old inner child who was stuck feeling unloved and lonely, as a result the adult Sunita was suffering in her relationships. After the deep introspection and self-realization, the 2 years old inner child was healed, and the adult Sunita was released from all the negative beliefs and emotions. After a year Sunita sent me a beautiful message to express her gratitude as her sinus was cured and visiting old buildings and monuments was no longer challenging.

**Healing Sinus:** You can refer to the healings of eyes, nasal and throat problems.

Chapter 9

# CHEST ISSUES

***"I do good to others but never get the same gesture back."***

## Lungs, Heart and Breast Issues

**Do you wonder, you keep doing so much for others but you do not get the same gesture back in return? Do you feel that when you need them, then they are not available to you? Do you feel that you go out of the way to help other people, but they feel that it was your duty and they never appreciate your efforts? Do people misunderstand you? Are you suffering from feelings of abandonment or fear of loneliness?**

Then you are at a high risk of experiencing chest pain, burning or other chest problems.

Major statements made by people suffering from chest issues:

*"I feel unloved."*

*"People take me for granted."*

*"People misunderstand me."*

*"People take advantage of me."*

*"I am scared of loneliness."*

*"I feel betrayed."*

*"People are jealous of me."*

*"I had been honest to this person always, but he/she broke my trust."*

Majority of my clients who reported chest problems experienced relationship conflicts. They ignored their own needs and devoted themselves to their loved ones completely. Such clients complained of chest issues like feeling heaviness in the chest or pressure, feeling like something stuck there.

Some people complained of slight recurrent pain that kept coming and going in their chest. They stated that according to the doctors, it could be gas that gets stuck or was revolving in the body because of their wrong eating habits. But that is not true. The primary root cause of chest problems is actually your relationship issues, conflicts or misunderstanding with your loved ones.

## LUNG PROBLEMS AND DISEASES: "It is my duty to take care of others."

### Asthma or Breathlessness:

The majority of my clients who complained of asthma or breathlessness issues confirmed a pattern of repeatedly taking on too many burdens of workloads. Most of them claimed that it was their environment that led them to helplessly take a lot of burdens. For instance, they were staying in a joint family and had no choice, or few said that they were divorced or separated and thus, had to handle everything on their own. However, in some cases there was a very strong fear of loneliness, and thus they kept themselves busy by taking on a lot of duties and work pressures. Most commonly felt emotions observed in such cases were anxiety, helplessness, fear of rejection and fear of loneliness.

### Case Study: Breathlessness, Anxiety, Acidity, Chest Pain

Michael, who was 26 years old, complained that when he ate food, he felt that it got stuck in his chest. He reported that this led to breathlessness, anxiety and restlessness and also sometimes, he felt dizzy and vomited. Since then, he developed a fear of eating food. Medically, doctors confirmed that he was absolutely fit, and thus, he was very anxious and worried, why was this happening, when all reports were fine. As a result, his work efficiency was affected, he could not focus on his job. He felt stuck in his situation which in turn increased his frustrations at job and intimate relationships. He said that he lost touch with friends and felt as if his life had come to an end. He continued to wonder why he had been suffering in all the spheres of his life, whether it was health, relationships and career. He went into depression and thus he consulted me for psychological counselling. He continued asking, "Why me? What have I done? Why am I suffering so much?"

Though his case included emotional turmoil symptoms, his physiological challenges needed to be addressed first, so Transpersonal regression therapy was executed to attain the greatest results. It was an unexpected past life session which beautifully connected to his current life. You will be absolutely startled as you read about what's unleashed a whirlwind of intense emotions and self-realization.

**Therapy Session:**

*Michael was so stressed that during the initial stage of conversation, he regressed into a deep trance state and the Hypnotherapy session began.*

*Therapist: "Imagine yourself eating food and tell me how you feel?"*

*After a long pause...*

*Client: "I am feeling anxious, food will get stuck..."*

*Therapist: "Any physical sensations?"*

*Client: "I am feeling heaviness in my chest and heart palpitations."*

*Therapist: "How is it making you feel?"*

*Client: "Something is stuck on my chest."*

*Therapist: "What is stuck on your chest?"*

*Client: "I don't know, I am feeling churning in my stomach."*

*Therapist: "What is happening?"*

*Client: "I am feeling dizzy, my head is spinning. I am feeling puckish. Jesus! I can't do this, I am feeling very uncomfortable, I am... I am stuck, I will die."*

*Therapist: "Where are you stuck, look around?"*

*Client: "It's a box, I am stuck, I can't breathe."*

*Therapist: "What are you feeling?"*

*Client: "I am feeling suffocated, my head is spinning. Oh my God! Oh shit! I can see, I am in a car. It toppled, it turned twice."*

*Therapist: "What is happening now?"*

*Client: "I am trying to open my belt. It's stuck, it's not opening."*

*Therapist: "How is it making you feel?"*

*Client: "I am panicking, I am feeling restless. I am not able to breathe, there is no one to help me. I am feeling helpless, I will die now."*

*Therapist: "Did you die there?"*

*Client: "Yes."*

*Therapist: "That life is now over."*

*Past life was healed and closed.*

*Therapist: "How are you feeling in your body, now?"*

*Client: "I am feeling better."*

*Therapist: "When did that past life trigger in your present life."*

*Client: "I was 22 years old."*

*Therapist: "What happened when you were 22 years old?"*

*Client: "I tested COVID positive."*

*Therapist: "What were you feeling at that time?"*

*Client: "I was stuck in one room for days, I could not breathe. I felt suffocated and restless as I was not allowed to go out of the room. I felt helpless. My anxiety kept on increasing when I thought, there is no one to help me and what will happen, if I die."*

*Therapist: "How long were you stuck there?"*

*Client: "For 25 days."*

*Therapist: "Were you fine after 25 days?"*

*Client: "Yes."*

*Therapist: "Any physical sensations right now?"*

*Client: "No sensations, I am feeling fine now."*

*The 22 years old inner child was healed and integrated with the 26 years old adult Michael and then the session was over.*

**Therapist Conclusion:**

After the therapy session, Michael consciously mentioned that when his mother came to stay with him a month back, they recalled their COVID memories and since then he started having the problem of heaviness in the chest and breathlessness. Actually, the memory of the COVID days triggered a past life in which he died with similar physical and emotional sensations such as breathlessness, restlessness, and helplessness that he had experienced while he was infected with COVID.

In his past life he was stuck in the car and felt breathlessness and anxiety because the belt did not open. Similarly in his current life, when he was 22 years old and infected with COVID, he was stuck in the small room and felt the same breathlessness and anxiety. It was the 22 years old inner child who was stuck in that moment feeling anxious and helpless. By recalling the COVID memories with his mother, all the traumatic emotions surfaced, and the 26 years old adult started suffering with the similar physical discomforts.

As mentioned in Chapter 1 "Health and Emotions", you can figure out the trigger of your health problem in your present, but the root cause of your problem always lies in your past.

By healing the 22 years old inner child, the adult Michael was released from all the physical sensations, uneasiness and pressures on his chest. After a few days, Michael testified and confirmed that he could eat food without any fear and did not feel breathlessness or heaviness in his chest. He also mentioned that before the session, he used to sometimes feel pain in left arm just near the shoulder blade, but after the session that pain was also healed.

**Case Study**: **Asthma, Breathlessness, Anxiety**

Hema, 36 years old, was struggling from asthma, shortness of breath, and throat congestion. It has gotten even worse with age. She claimed that it worsened during the winter season and could not find any solution to her problem. her anxiety increased further as she developed fear of death. Thus, she decided to take psychological help to heal her anxiety and fear of death. Transpersonal Regression was executed for the instant results; it was an unexpected and mind-blowing session that culminated in an avalanche of unbelievable insights that will leave you perplexed as it unfolds. Her case study is a perfect example that is going to demonstrate you how a single regression therapy session can heal not only emotional symptoms but also physiological disorders without the use of medicine.

**Therapy Session:**

*Hema was induced a deep Hypnotic state and the therapy session began.*

*Therapist: "When do you feel more breathless, any particular time in the day or always?"*

*Client: "When I take a bath, I feel more."*

*Therapist: "When you feel breathless how does it make you feel?"*

*Client: "I feel very anxious and very helpless. I feel I will die?"*

*Therapist: "Imagine yourself taking a bath, what are you feeling?"*

*Client: "I am feeling anxious."*

*Client starts breathing heavily.*

*Therapist: "Any physical sensations?"*

*Client: "Heart palpitation, I am feeling dizzy. I am getting chills."*

*Therapist: "What do you mean by chills?"*

*Client: "I am getting goosebumps, my hands and feet are freezing. I can't breathe, I am feeling suffocated. I am stuck, water will kill me, please take me out! I beg you, please take me out!"*

*Client started crying out loudly.*

*Therapist: "Where are you?"*

*Client: "I am in a small room or a cabin, it's very dark, everything is falling down. I am trying to open the room door, it's not opening. I can hear noise of people outside the door, they are banging the door, asking me to open, but its stuck. I am feeling very scared."*

*Therapist: "What is happening?"*

*Client: "I can feel water coming into the room from the edge of the door. Yes, I think, I am in a ship, it's sinking. Oh my God! I am feeling puckish, it's very suffocating, water is rising, oh my God! My body is freezing, my feet have become numb. I am stuck, I can't breathe, I will die now."*

*Client cried out loudly as she started choking due to which breathlessness increased.*

*Therapist: "Did you die there?"*

*Client: "Yes."*

*Therapist: "Just make a mental note, THAT LIFE IS NOW OVER."*

*The healing was done, and the client was made comfortable. Then the session continued...*

*Therapist: "When did that past life trigger in your current life?"*

*Client: "I was 25 years old."*

*Therapist: "What happened when you were 25 years old?"*

*Client: "I went to Nainital, I sat on the boat with my husband, I was very happy."*

*Therapist: "What happened on the boat that made you feel anxious and helpless?"*

*Client: "I remember, I was very excited. I tried to stand on the boat to click pictures. I moved from one side of the boat to another due to which the boat starting shaking, and got disbalanced, the person who was rowing the boat, started shouting. I got very scared by his loud voice, I felt confused. I went blank for some time and started feeling dizzy and puckish. We immediately returned back."*

*After listening to the story, the 25 years old inner child of Hema was healed and integrated with the adult.*

*Therapist: "Are you feeling any physical sensations now?"*

*Client: "No, I'm feeling fine now."*

*Therapist: "When you are comfortable, open your eyes."*

**Therapist Conclusion:**

After the therapy session, Hema mentioned consciously that when she was born, she had no phobias of water bodies, nor did she have any breathing or throat problems. However, after the boat incident when she was 25 years old, she began to experience dizziness near bodies of water, which led to anxiety, heart palpitations, and shortness of breath. This worsened over time and led to her being diagnosed with asthma.

Actually, when Hema was in the boat and it shook, the rower started shouting. She got extremely frightened and her memory of the past life in which she died in the water feeling the same destruction, noise and physical sensations, got triggered. It was the 25 years old inner child who was stuck in past memory. Although after coming out of the boat 36 years old adult Hema was absolutely fine. But the 25 years old inner child remained frozen at that moment and thus, the adult was suffering since then. By healing the inner child, the adult was liberated from the past traumatic memory. It was the most unexpected and unforgettable therapy session I'd ever had at work.

After observing herself for a period of 3 months, she testified that she didn't feel fear of water anymore. Moreover, her breathlessness was also cured, and she was out of inhalers.

**Other Lung diseases:**

Clients who suffered from water accumulation in the lungs showed a repeated pattern of being stuck in the past hurtful memories which involved their parents, siblings, children or spouse. They felt guilty for failing in playing their roles as it was expected from them. Most of them displayed feelings of guilt and helplessness.

**Lung cancer:**

It was observed that most of the clients suffering from lung cancer, displayed a lot of resentment, anger, loneliness, guilt. The majority of them admitted that they experienced separation anxiety when they were distant from their loved ones. As you continue reading, you will have a greater understanding of this through a beautiful case study that involved intense catharsis and deep healing at both physical as well as emotional level.

**Case Study: Lung Cancer**

One of my clients suffering from lung cancer, in her Hypnotherapy session, regressed to her childhood in time where she pointed out issues with her siblings. She was the eldest and loved them a lot, but she felt that they did not love her in the same way. Being the eldest, she felt that it was her responsibility to take care of them and she selflessly looked after them, but when they behaved selfishly with her, she used to get angry. However, she never expressed her anger and instead helplessly kept on nurturing them.

Although she consciously felt love for them, she was subconsciously very angry, sad and wounded at heart. She could never forgive them, and the resentment built deep within her. The emotions that she felt deeply were resentment, anxiety, loneliness, guilt and helplessness. Through the therapy session she released all her unwavering negative emotions and beliefs that led to cancer. The most important part of the session that led to i healing was the cathartic moment and exquisite self-realisation which was extremely essential to stop the cancer from spreading.

Cancer does not emerge overnight or suddenly; it is caused by subconsciously suppressed permeating painful emotions that consume you like termites. Deep cleansing of your subconscious mind is the most vital step towards faster recovery from cancer.

**Healing Lung Issues:**

To heal your lung issues, first take a deep breathe. Find moments of stillness or silence within yourself. Focus on yourself and avoid taking burdens of responsibilities. This does not mean that you have to ignore your duties and sit idle. You have to acknowledge your responsibilities but complete your tasks in your capacity. You don't have to prove yourself to anyone. You don't have to seek approval from others. You are both your own attorney and your own judge. Appreciate yourself and others unconditionally. You are both a critic and an admirer. Liberate yourself from the fear of losing your loved ones. Remember on Earth, if you have karmic teachers, who give you bitterness, then you have soul connections also, who shower you with love and blessings. Just make peace within that everyone is there for you. You don't have to work hard to make them yours. What is yours will always be yours. Whoever loves you will always love you. You don't have to go the extra mile to impress everyone.

Practice gratitude as well as positive thoughts. Forgive yourself and other people. Let go of your past through deep introspection and gain wisdom with positive understanding.

Chakras: If you are suffering from lung diseases, then it implies that your throat chakra, heart chakra and the solar plexus chakra may be either partially blocked or completely blocked. Take charge of your life. Don't feel guilty and stop punishing yourself. Accept yourself the way you are. Understand your limitations and boundaries. Listen to your breath and talk to your inner self. It is fine to say, “No” if it is beyond your mark. You don't have to go out of the way to please anybody. Clear communication is very important. You can politely express your sentiments and point of views to other people. To activate your throat chakra, heart chakra, and the solar plexus chakra, you can refer to the chakra section in this book.

**Affirmations:**

*"I take responsibilities in my capacity."*

*"I love and accept myself as I am."*

## HEART PROBLEMS:
## "I feel people take advantage of my goodness."

**Do you wonder why the people you love the most hurt you the most? Do you believe you do good for others, yet they frequently misinterpret you? Do you believe that others take advantage of your goodness? Are you the victim of a backstab?**

Then proceed with caution, as your heart may be in danger of problems like high blood pressures, heart attack, heart failure, arrhythmia, valve disease, sinus tachycardia etc. Heart is the symbol of love. People who suffer from heart problems are empathetic, they love and trust people easily and quickly. They suffer as a result of their high expectations from other people, which are frequently not met. They feel constantly frustrated, disappointed, unloved, lonely, and resentful throughout their lives.

Most of my clients who suffered from heart conditions felt very lonely as they lost their loved ones to death or faced betrayals from their loved ones, including their relatives, and especially siblings. They were unable to forgive them and continued to replay past traumatic memories in their minds, which increased their stress and strong feelings of grudges, hatred and sorrow. Clients with heart problems also displayed a strong *fear of the unknown* that was the major cause of their high blood pressures.

**Case Study**

Anil who was 56 years old had suffered from a heart attack at age 47 and had developed fear of death and wanted to deal with it. During his counselling session, he told me that his younger brother had betrayed him in business. They were jointly running a family business and his younger brother took care of all the paperwork while he used to take care of the field work. His younger brother took all the bank loans in Anil's name and Anil, who blindly trusted his brother, didn't have any clue of his malice intentions and used to sign all the documents without reading them. He was shocked, when he was asked to repay the large sum of the bank loan in 1 month. He was bankrupt, he had to sell his house to repay the loan. He also mentioned that his son had enrolled for higher studies abroad, but could not go after that incident. His son also blamed him for being foolish. Anil felt guilty and helpless. After about 6 months, he suddenly fainted and experienced a heart attack. Anil cried, "I loved my brother so much and I always did good to him, then why did he betray me, what did I do?" The shocking revelation of the root cause of Anil's heart attack will leave you perplexed. As you read his story, you will discover how deep introspection of your own subconscious mind during the session clears the large dark cloud of false beliefs and illusions that you forged. This incredible session will help you understand that you are a victim of your own thoughts and limiting beliefs.

**Therapy Session:**

*During the Hypnotherapy session Anil regressed to his age of 5. In the trance session, he said that he used to feel that his mother loved the younger brother more than him and thus he would feel jealous of him. He went back in time to the moment when his brother, who was 1.5 years old, was sleeping. Anil out of jealousy and anger pushed him off the bed. When his mother heard the child crying, she ran towards him. She picked him up into her arms and started kissing him.*

*Anil was very happy after throwing the child, but became very angry when saw his mother's love for his younger brother. Mother scolded Anil and told him that he was the elder brother, so it was his responsibility to take care of his younger brother. She forced the 5 years old Anil, to take the oath to always love his younger brother and be there for him at all times. Anil was very angry in heart, but loved his mother very much and thus he helplessly took the oath. Since then, he tried to love his brother only consciously, but he developed a lot of anger towards him subconsciously.*

Self-realization and wisdom was gained by Anil as healing of the 5 years old inner child was completed. Adult Anil understood the reason for why his brother betrayed him. He forgave his brother and was released from the rage, resentment and sorrow that he had been carrying in his heart for so many years.

**Therapist Conclusion:**

Anil had taken the oath to love his brother only because he loved his mother, but within his heart he carried a lot of grudges towards his younger brother. As they grew old, Anil had consciously forgotten everything and tried to genuinely love his brother and be good to him. However, his brother's behaviour was a subconscious reflection of suppressed anger and resentment that Anil was carrying since childhood towards him. Through the beautiful self-realization, everything became transparent like a mirror, and he understood how his negative emotions were deflected back by his brother towards him. The ultimate source of all complexity within their relationship was the 5 years old inner child of Anil who was stuck in the past feeling poisoned emotions.

**Guidance:** Other people's actions are nothing but your subconscious reflections. If you feel others are not being good with you or betray you, then that implies you are carrying certain negative beliefs or suppressed emotions that are being reflected back to you. For instance, if you feel people judge you, paradoxically this means that you are judgmental; you have a subconscious tendency to judge people. If you perceive that people are not understanding you then this means you are unable to understand others.

Life will become simple if you remember that the other person is only mirroring you. Focus on your triggered emotions rather than other people's actions. Don't suppress your unwavering thoughts and emotions by pretending to be good. No doubt you are a good person, but your repressed emotions belong to your traumatic past which is creating chaos in your present. Not only your health, but also your relationships and finances are at stake. You just need to heal these emotions to lead a fulfilling life.

**Blood Pressure:** High or low blood pressures are caused due to stress and bitterness in a relationship. You may be taking over burdens and responsibilities of work, multitasking, but you feel that your loved ones never appreciate you, rather always misunderstand you or take you for granted.

**Do you wonder that outwardly, you are a fun loving bubbly kind of a person, who likes to enjoy life and doesn't take things to heart? Are you one of those who doesn't care what other people are saying or thinking about you?**

Ironically, people around you matter! You are very sensitive at heart. You care for other people and feel hurt when they do not reciprocate in the same way. As you read the next case study, you will understand the root cause of high blood pressure.

**Case Study:** High blood pressure and increased heart rate.

Vinay, 42, had been suffering from high blood pressure problems for the past 3 years. He reported that despite being on medicine, his blood pressure remained elevated. He told me that when he got up in the morning, his heart rate used to be 250 beats per minute, despite the fact that 72 beats per minute is what is considered normal. So, he wanted to take Regression therapy to heal his problems. It was a staggering session which involved beautiful inner child healing and enormous release of carmine emotions.

**Therapy Session:**

Vinay was induced a deep trance state and the therapy session commenced.

*Therapist: "Go to the last moment when your heartbeat was very high."*

*Client: "I see myself on the road and I am not able to walk to the car which is so near to me."*

*Therapist: "What are you feeling?"*

*Client: "I am feeling stuck, I can't move."*

*Therapist: "Any physical sensations?"*

*Client: "Yes, I am feeling heaviness in my heart."*

*Therapist: "What is this heaviness making you feel."*

*Client: "I feel that something will happen to me. I feel trapped. I can't breathe. There is no one to help me. I feel, I will die."*

*Therapist: "Where are you trapped, look around?"*

*Client: "It is a small room."*

*Therapist: "How old are you?"*

*Client: "I am 7 years old."*

*Therapist: "What happened when you were 7 years old?"*

*Client: "My mother locked me in the room because I had a fight with my sibling."*

*Therapist: "How did you feel at that moment?"*

*Client: "Oh! I got so scared, I felt trapped in that room. I kept banging the door, but she didn't open it."*

*Therapist: "What did you feel when she didn't open the door?"*

*Client: "I felt extremely angry because she was very impartial towards me. She loved my younger brother more than me."*

*Therapist: "Why do you feel that she was impartial towards you?"*

*Client: "I kept on explaining, but she never listened to me. She always held me responsible when there were any fights between me and my sibling."*

*Therapist: "How did that make you feel?"*

*Client: "I felt unsupported and unloved. I felt I had to stand for myself. No one was there for me."*

*Client started feeling pain in his left arm.*

*Therapist: "For how long were you locked in that room?"*

*Client: "For about 2 hours."*

*After telling the story, the 7 years old inner child was healed.*

*Therapist: "Do you feel any pain in your left arm or heaviness in your heart now?"*

*Client: "No."*

*Session was then ended.*

**Therapist Conclusion:**

Through the insightful therapy session, it was concluded that Vinay, the adult, felt stuck and trapped because his 7 years old inner child had been frozen in the painful memory of his mother locking him in the room. The inner child felt scared and unloved, and he was angry at his mother because he believed she was impartial towards him. However, after the session the 42 years old adult Vinay consciously stated that he is now a father of 2 children and understands that parents love their children equally. It was the 7 years old inner child Vinay who felt that his mother didn't understand him and continually blamed him for everything.

After a month, Vinay reported that his heart rate was absolutely normal when he woke up in the morning, and his blood pressure was also likewise normal. I often gave his example to most of my clients who were stuck on questions like "Why me?" The amazing discoveries of his session and the remarkable outcome have given answers to so many clients and healed them at conscious level.

Heart problems or chest pains occur when there are suppressed past emotions of sadness or resentment over your loved ones during your childhood. These emotions remain dormant in your subconscious mind without affecting you much, but whenever in your current situation face a similar type of issue with your loved ones then those repressed emotions resurface and lead to heartache. This heart ache is an initial signal of the triggered past emotions and should be tackled in time. Medication can only heal your physical, it cannot heal your tumultuous emotions. You can avoid major heart problems if you seek emotional counselling and heal your suppressed emotions.

**Healing Heart Problems:**

Transpersonal Regression therapy, Hypnotherapy or relationship counselling are the most effective ways to heal your heart issues. These therapy sessions help you to contemplate your past situations through an adult view and brings self-realization. The deep introspection and awareness sheds new light on the adult perspective which helps you to let go of your past and forgive other people easily.

Heart chakra activation is essential to heal your heart problems. You have to learn to give and receive unconditional love. Avoid expectations. Feel love and compassion for others. Build trust on self and other people. Along with the heart chakra, throat chakra and the solar plexus chakra also gets imbalanced. Take charge of life. Don't suppress your emotions. Communicate clearly and express your feelings and needs.

Refer to the chakra section to learn about this in detail.

Liberate yourself from your wounded past. Let the scars in your heart heal with divine wisdom and understanding. Before taking birth on Earth, it was you who chose these people to complete your learnings. You are the director of the entire play, and everyone who enters into your life is simply performing the role that you have assigned to them. Practice forgiveness, positive thinking and attitude. Express gratitude and thanksgiving to even non-living things. Spread love unconditionally.

**Affirmations:**

*"I love and accept myself."*

*"I give and accept love unconditionally."*

*"I forgive myself and others."*

*"I release myself and (person's name) from the obligation of teaching lessons to each other."*

Avoid stress and remain calm. You can do yoga, physical exercises and emotion management techniques (you can find them in the healing section of the book). Heart chakra takes its energy from greenery, so just take a nature walk and breathe in fresh air with a positive mindset.

Do meditation to heal and balance your heart chakra and other chakras. You can refer to the meditation given under the healing section of the book. This meditation will help you to forgive people who left you with a wounded heart and improve your sleep patterns.

## BREAST PROBLEMS:
## "My family is my priority."

**Are you one of those who ignores yourself and has devoted yourself completely to your loved ones or people around you?**

If yes, then you may be at a risk of suffering from breast issues like breast pain or tenderness, stiffness, cysts, lumps, boils, nipple discharge or inversion, fibroadenomas, fat necrosis, gynecomastia, breast cancer, etc. Following is a beautiful past life regression case study that will help you to understand how only nurturing others and ignoring thyself can be devastating.

**Case study: Breast lumps**

Soni, who was 45 years old, had been suffering from lumps in her left breast for the past 3 years. She reported to me that doctors gave her antibiotics for 7 days and she felt better, but the lumps returned after a few months. So, she was worried as to why the problem persisted. Moreover, she had a family history of breast cancer as her mother and grandmother both suffered from the disease. Thus, each time she felt pain in her breast and lumps formed, she used to feel very anxious. Therefore, she decided to tap into the root cause of the problem through the Hypnotherapy session and heal it. It was a lovely session in which she discovered that the root cause of her suffering lay dormant in her past life and had a remarkable impact on her present life. You'll be taken aback when you stumble upon her story of how her past life emotions rebounded in her current life, leaving her befuddled. It will help you to understand how your current life relationship issues can trigger the memories of your deeply suppressed past life events and cause physical symptoms in your current life.

**Therapy Session:**

*During the session, she told me that she used to feel very lonely. Her husband used to travel a lot and they lived in a nuclear family. She had issues with both her parents and siblings. She did not have any friends, so she devoted all her time to her son who was 17 years old. As she started talking about her son, her body language changed and she regressed into a deep trance state.*

*Therapist: "What is happening?"*

*Client: "I am feeling pain in my left breast."*

*Therapist: "Tap into this pain, describe it, how is making you feel?"*

*Client: "I am feeling as if someone is pricking needles in my body."*

*Therapist: "How does it make you feel?"*

*Client: "I feel angry and helpless."*

*Therapist: "How old are you?"*

*Client: "I am 67 years old."*

*It was evident, Client regressed to her past life, as in her current life, she was just 45 years old.*

*Therapist: "Where are you?"*

*Client: "I live in a very big house, I have 3 sons who are married and have children. We all stay together in a joint family. We are very rich and we have many servants."*

*Therapist: "Go to the next important moment in that lifetime."*

*Client cried out loudly: "I am feeling a lot of pain in my breast."*

*Therapist: "How did you die in that lifetime?"*

*Client: "I had breast cancer."*

*Therapist: "Be in the last moment, just before you die, see it in slow motion. Where are you? Who is there with you?"*

*Client cried: "I am in my room and no one is there with me."*

*Therapist: "Where is everyone?"*

*Client: "They are busy in their own lives, they don't have time for me. No one needs me, everyone is so... selfish."*

*Therapist: "Why do you feel they are selfish?"*

*Client: "They don't love me, they come to me only when they need money from me."*

*Therapist: "How does it make you feel as you are dying, and no one is there?"*

*Client: "I feel very angry. Oh! I am so alone, I feel so helpless, no one is there for me."*

*Therapist: "Now, that life is over."*

*The past life was healed with all the necessary closures and then the session was continued.*

*Therapist: "Soni, see that age of you when that past life got triggered in your current life? How old are you?"*

*Client: "I am 38 years old?"*

*Therapist: "What is the 38 years old Soni feeling?"*

*Client: "I am feeling very sad and lonely, my husband keeps traveling due to work and my son has no time for me. He keeps confined to his own room. He does not even let me enter his room. I try to keep myself busy by cooking new dishes for my son, but he doesn't care about anything. He comes to me only when he needs food and money. I feel like I am just an ATM for him, nothing else.*

*Therapist: "How does that make you feel?"*

*Client: "I feel very angry and irritated over him, but he is my son, I can't do anything about it?"*

The client's body language changed. She started feeling pain in her feet and fingers.

The physical pains and the negative emotions were healed along with integration… towards the end of such an intense session, all the physical sensations were rechecked from the client.

*Therapist: "Are you still having any pains?"*

*Client: "No, I am fine."*

*Therapist: "So, you can open your eyes, when you feel comfortable."*

**Therapist Conclusion:**

It was clear from the therapy session that when Soni was 38 years old, she started feeling very lonely as her husband had to travel due to work and her 17 years old son didn't take care of her. After the session she consciously confirmed that the pains in her breast started during that age only. She told me that when her son was young, she used to spend all her time with him, but when he turned 10 years of age, he started distancing himself from her. He became very rude and was always irritated with her. She tried to take care of him, but his behaviour pushed them apart. He only came to her when he needed money for expensive watches and gadgets. She felt very angry, lonely and helpless.

Since in her past life, she suffered a similar situation and died feeling the same emotions, that past life got triggered. As a result, all the associated breast pains experienced in that lifetime also surfaced, when she was 38 years old. The 38 years old inner child of Soni was healed and the adult 45 years old Soni was liberated from her traumatic past episodes. After one year, Soni emailed to me and confirmed that she did not feel any pains or lumps in her breast. She told me that she had started her own fashion boutique and was feeling very happy and satisfied in her life.

Closures are very important to lead a healthy and fulfilling life because if you get stuck in a negative thought process, then all unwavering emotions get triggered due to which all the past painful memories resurface and add to your misery. Then you feel miserable in every sphere of your life, health, finances and relationships. Therefore, a healthy mindset is the key to a healthy lifestyle and there should be a proper balance of love. You can love others, but love yourself in the same way. If you feel that you love yourself but still you are suffering from breast issues, then the primary root cause of your problem lies deep in your past; it could be childhood or past lifetime.

**Do you know the emotional reasons for the pain in Left Breast and Right Breast are different?**

After the detailed study on all my clients who came with breast issues, I observed that the **Left breast** gets affected if you are facing issues with your children. Most of my clients who suffered with lumps or cysts, boils and cancer in their left breast, carried a lot of anger and resentment towards their children. While the problems in the **Right breast** seemed to be caused due to external factors like problems with the spouse or other people in your immediate environment. They carried a lot of grudges and resentment towards their spouse, siblings and in-laws.

**Healing Breast Issues:**

Practice self-love. Accept and love yourself just as you are. Learn to set aside time for yourself. It is absolutely fine to love and care for yourself in the same way as you love and care for others in your family. It is critical to recognise oneself. Do not disregard your own needs.

Do things in your capacity for your loved ones and do not expect anything in return. Give unconditional love. Address issues with your children and spouse. Try to learn from them. They are teaching you some important lessons of life that would be beneficial for you. They are your reflections, they will mirror you. For example, if your child is getting irritated, then it is you who is feeling irritated in your life. You just need to heal your irritation. Talk to yourself and ask, "Why are you feeling irritated?"

Shadow work is a deep inner child healing work; it helps you to look within and discover the root cause of your issues in life. It assists you in understanding your true self and heals you quickly. It aids in faster recovery from the issues of your breast as well as heals your relationship with your children, spouse and siblings.

Heart Chakra Activation: Breast is a part of the heart chakra, so you can heal the Breast issues by activating your heart chakra in the following ways:

**1. Nature**: Heart chakra takes its energy from nature. Thus, it can be activated by spending time in open space, in parks, gardens or hills.

**2. Self-love**: Self-love is the key to heal your chest problems. By practicing self-love, you can feel peace within you. It helps you to fill up all the voids and value yourself.

*Do you know the difference between self-love and selfishness?*

Self-love entails loving oneself as well as being empathetic towards others. Taking care of yourself while also meeting the needs and desires of others.

Selfishness is defined as solely loving oneself without concern for others. When you are willing to go to any extent to profit oneself without regard for how it may affect others.

**3. Affirmations:**

*"I love myself."*

*"I accept myself as I am."*

*"I feel safe to trust people."*

*"I do good to others and good comes back to me in the same way."*

*"I understand people and people understand me."*

**4. Chakras:** The throat chakra and the solar plexus chakra also get imbalanced along with heart chakra when you are suffering from breast issues. When you are not able to communicate clearly with your children or your life partner, then you probably suffer from breast issues. As a result, throat chakra and the heart chakra start getting imbalanced. Solar plexus chakra is the chakra of control. When you feel loss of control in your life then solar plexus chakra gets blocked either partially or completely. Majority of the cases who were suffering from breast issues displayed a very strong fear of loss of control in their life with their spouse and children. Learn about these chakras in detail under the chakra section.

Chest issues occur when you have relationship and thus, it is essential to keep in mind that if you do not understand the root cause of your chest pains and heal the triggered repressed emotions, then it can lead to other health issues affecting your stomach, liver, kidneys, joint pains, urinary infections or diabetes. As you will read further you will be able to understand how relationships conflict and affect your health.

# *Chapter 10*
# ABDOMINAL PAINS AND DISEASES

***"I feel stuck and helpless."***

## STOMACH ISSUES AND INTESTINES:
## "I get stuck in why? What? And when?"

**Do you feel stuck in a loop of endless negative thoughts or overthinking?**

If your mind is constantly overthinking or you keep dwelling into negative thoughts, then you are bound to struggle with stomach issues like acidity, gas, stomach cramps, constipation or loose motion, Irritable Bowel Syndrome, diarrhoea, swelling in small intestines or anal problems, etc.

Do you know where your mind is physically located in your body?

Mind is a ball of energy all around you and the source of this energy is your abdomen, solar plexus chakra. As you will read further, you will understand about chakras in detail. Yes, your mind is the energy that originates from your abdomen, therefore, whenever there is clogging of too many thoughts in your mind due to overthinking, then your abdomen gets affected. Have you ever noticed, when you are struggling with your finances, career or even in relationships, then you experience stomach problems?

Being too logical or analytical, taking excess work pressures or relationship conflicts causes anxiety and a lot of stress, which in turn leads to stomach issues. As mentioned earlier, stress releases hormones like cortisol and adrenaline which makes your mind hyperactive. Excess secretion of these hormones, consequently, upsets your stomach. And this is also one of the reasons why you experience stomach issues, when you have exams or job interviews. In short, it is your mind and thought processes that create your health problems.

Not only thoughts, but your emotions also lead to clogging of your mind, which lead to various health issues and diseases. Do you have a habit of holding yourself responsible for everything that goes wrong around you? Always feeling guilty for your actions leads to gas, acidity, cramps and stomach pains. Guilt is stored as self-anger in your subconscious mind. Some people consciously feel guilty and keep criticizing themselves. Self-criticism leads to stomach problems. Further, when there is a lot of bitterness in your wounded heart for someone, you have a tendency to dwell into the past and you are not able to let go. You constantly, keep thinking about your past traumatic events and people who gave you those pains. Then this leads to clogging of your mind, consequently you suffer from constipation.

**What is Constipation?**

Constipation in literal sense implies you are trying to hold too much in your body and unable to release it. It is actually the thoughts and suppressed emotions that you are holding on to, due to which you suffer from constipation.

Statements, generally made by people who struggle with constipation:

*"I feel stuck in life."*

*"My finances are stuck."*

*"My career is stuck."*

*"My job is at stake."*

*"I have deadlines to meet."*

*"I am stressed about my exams."*

*"I want to remember all the concepts till my exam is over."*

Constipation occurs when you feel stuck in life. When you are scared of moving ahead in life. As a result, you feel stagnant at one place. Your mind feels stuck.

It is also observed through my case studies, that when there is too much holding back of past grudges, blame and constant replaying of the traumatic memories, you suffer from constipation. I observed that when I told such clients to let go of the past then they all started following statements:

*"I have forgotten everything."*

*"All that was in the past."*

*"It's okay, I have now moved on."*

*"I don't even remember anything now."*

It is important for you to understand that your mind never forgets anything. Even if you suffer from amnesia or any memory loss diseases, your subconscious keeps your traumatic memories stored. These memories keep triggering and all your, unhealed emotions resurface, causing health problems like stomach issues, swelling in small intestines or large intestine issues, etc.

For instance, there was a client Sharda, 58 years old, who wished to seek Regression therapy to treat her acidity, gas and constipation issues that lead to swelling in her small intestines. The unexpected disclosure and the way the whole therapy session unfolded will deeply touch your soul.

**Case Study:**

The Hypnotherapy session began after a few breathing exercises and relaxation.

*Therapist: "Are you feeling acidity or any discomfort now?"*

*Client: "No, I take medicine in the morning, so it's fine right now."*

*Therapist: "So when you feel stomach discomfort, then how does that make you feel?"*

*Client: "I feel burning in my stomach, sometimes nausea and headache."*

*Therapist: "How does that make you feel?"*

*Client: "I feel anxious. I keep figuring out, what did I eat that has led to this pain?"*

*Therapist: "How does that make you feel?"*

*Client: "I feel very angry, irritated and helpless."*

*Therapist: "Feel this anxiety, anger, irritation and helplessness growing, as you think, why is this happening to me?"*

*Client became uncomfortable and started choking.*

*Therapist: "What is happening to you?"*

*Client: "I am feeling burning in my stomach and something is choking in my throat."*

*Therapist: "What is choking in your throat?"*

*Client said anxiously: "I feel it's smoke; yes, it's smoke."*

*Therapist: "Where are you?"*

*Client: "I am in the kitchen."*

*Therapist: "What is happening in the kitchen?"*

*Client suddenly folded her hands, her body squeezed inwards.*

*Client started screaming: "I see smoke all around, I have caught fire."*

*Therapist: "What happened?"*

*Client became silent. After a long pause, the session continued.*

*Therapist: "What happened next?"*

*Client: "I died... I can see my dead body on the floor."*

*Client regressed to her past life.*

*Therapist: "Just go back to a few moments, before you die. Tell me, how did you catch fire?"*

*Client: "I burnt myself."*

*Therapist: "Why?"*

*Client: "I was feeling very angry over my husband; he had an extramarital affair. So, I committed suicide."*

*Therapist: "As you were committing suicide, what were your thoughts?"*

*Client: "I felt why did this happen to me? What was my mistake?"*

*Therapist: "Okay, so now that life is over."*

*Past life was healed and closures were done.*

*Therapist: "When did that past life trigger in your current life? Take an impression, how old are you?"*

*Client: "I am 5 years old, it is my birthday party."*

*Therapist: "What happened in your birthday party that made you feel angry."*

*Client: "I remember that when I bent down to blow the candles, I saw that my aunt was holding my sister in her arms."*

*Therapist: "What did this make you feel?"*

*Client: "I felt very angry?"*

*Therapist: "Over whom, were you angry?"*

*Client: "On my sister."*

*Therapist: "Why?"*

*Client: "Everyone loved her. Since she was born, my mother also cared for her more than me. She just had forgotten me as if I didn't exist. It was my birthday, but everyone was asking for my sister and playing with her, and not me."*

*Therapist: "How did this make you feel?"*

*Client: "I felt so angry and so rejected. I used to feel what was my mistake? Why does my mother love my sister more? I kept wondering, maybe I was dark in complexion and my sister was fair, so my mother loved her more."*

*Therapist: "Do you still feel this?"*

*Client: "No, no, absolutely not. As I am a mother of two kids now, I understand that for parents all children are equal. My sister was one year old at that time, that is why, my mother had to take care of her more, and everyone played with her because she was an infant. Obviously, people play with infants more, I realize that now."*

*After the beautiful self-realization by the adult, the 5 years old inner child was healed and integrated.*

*Therapist: "Any discomfort in your stomach or throat?"*

*Client: "No, it's fine now."*

*Therapist: "How are you feeling now?"*

*Client: "I feel very peaceful and satisfied. Thank you!"*

*Then the heart touching session ended.*

**Therapist Conclusion:**

Through the therapy session it was concluded that the 5 years old inner child was stuck in the past, feeling angry and rejected. When the 5 years old Sharda bent down to blow the candles and saw the fire, suddenly her past life in which she burnt herself got triggered, and thus, all the emotions associated with that lifetime surfaced. In her previous life, she felt angry and rejected by her husband, and thus, committed suicide. She died thinking, "Why did this happen to me? What was my mistake?"

Similarly, in this lifetime, when her mother loved her sister more than her, she thought the same. Consequently, her anger, jealousy and feelings of rejection led to stomach issues with her increasing age. Later, when she suffered with acidity and gas pain. She again thought the same, "What did I eat that led to this pain? Why can't I eat like other people?" These thoughts amplified her emotions of anger, irritation and feeling of helplessness due to which she suffered.

After the session, she told me that she felt rejected even after her marriage by her mother-in-law, as she was dark in complexion and her mother-in- law wanted a daughter in law with fair complexion. It was very clear that due to the past life trigger, her traumatic emotions kept amplifying and she continued drawing negative conclusions about herself. Consequently, a loop was created in her subconscious mind, as a result of which, she kept attracting similar events, which made her feel more angry and more rejected. She tried to be good to others, but the goodness was not reciprocated in the same way which led to a lot of anger on self. She felt guilty for being so good with others. This in turn led to more frustrations, and thus, she suffered with intense stomach issues.

Therefore, in order to heal your stomach, it's important to take charge of your thoughts and emotions. After the healing session, Sharda was cured from her traumatic past memories. She understood how her past was impacting her present and creating chaotic emotions. Regression therapy can only help you heal your past and become aware of the primary cause of your problem. Sharda's constipation and stomach problems were completely cured after the healing session, but it was now her job to maintain check of her thoughts and emotions in the future, or the stomach issues would reoccur.

Your health issues in future, entirely depend on your thought process. You have to maintain a healthy mindset for a healthy living else a stuck mindset will make you feel stuck in life. Your health, finances and relationships, in every sphere of your life will find yourself STUCK.

When you are under extreme pressure or stress or when you are stuck in a "What if?" situation, feeling terribly scared or going through a period of uncertainty, then you are subconsciously feeling a lot of anxiety and fear of the unknown, which can also cause stomach upset or loose motions.

If you have to make important decisions in life which could affect your future, then failures in your past decisions may trigger the fear in you. Thus, you dwell into overthinking. A part of you wants to move ahead with the decision but there is another part of you that feels horrified.

This inner conflict leads to stomach upset and you may experience loose motions also.

For instance, Manish, who was 56 years old, suddenly started experiencing stomach cramps, loose motions, dizziness and vomiting. Doctors suspected diarrhoea, but all his blood tests were absolutely normal. His health was driving him crazy. Completely puzzled and confused Manish then finally decided to seek psychotherapy counselling to heal himself. It was an amazing session, and the outcome will leave you awestruck. It will help you comprehend how minor disagreements and stress in your present may stir up profoundly suppressed emotions from your past, which can have a huge impact on your health.

**Case Study**

Manish was induced a deep hypnotic state and the therapy session began.

*Therapist: "Are you having any physical discomforts right now?"*

*Client: "No, I am on antibiotics, so I feel better now. But I am scared that after 2 days my antibiotics course will end, and then again I will suffer from stomach cramps and loose motions."*

*Therapist: "Why do you feel so if medication is healing you?"*

*Client: "Few days before also, doctors prescribed me antibiotics, I was fine only till I continued the medication. All the symptoms relapsed after I stopped the medication."*

*Therapist: "How does this thought make you feel?"*

*Client: "Oh! I'm very anxious and confused. I feel so helpless and trapped. My mind constantly keeps bugging me with thoughts like what should I do? What is going to happen now? How long will I be stuck in this? Will I ever recover?"*

*Therapist: "Feel this anxiety, this confusion, helplessness as you are trapped."*

*Client started feeling restless and started pressing his stomach.*

*Therapist: "What is happening?"*

*Client: "I am feeling stomach ache, heaviness in my legs and giddiness."*

*Therapist: "Feel this heaviness in your legs, how does it make you feel?"*

*Client: "I feel as if, something heavy is on my leg, so I can't move my legs, I feel stuck"*

*Therapist: "How does this make you feel?"*

*Client: "I am feeling so scared and confused. What is happening?*

*Therapist: "Go back in time to the moment, when you felt so scared and confused, feeling trapped as if something very heavy was on your legs and you could not move."*

*After a long pause the session continued.*

*Therapist: "Where are you?"*

*Client: "I am blank."*

*Therapist: "Is it light or darkness?"*

*Client: "It's light."*

*Therapist: "Where is this light?"*

*Client: "I am stuck under a big stone, I can't move. My whole body is stuck."*

*Therapist: "Just go back a few moments, before this, how did you get stuck there?"*

*Client started feeling dizzy.*

*Therapist: "What is happening?*

*Client: "My head is spinning, everything around me is also spinning."*

*Therapist: "Where are you?"*

*Client: "I can feel like an earthquake is coming, I am on the bed and it suddenly started shaking. Everything is falling down, I can see cracks on the ceiling, lights have broken and the floor is shaking."*

Client regressed to his past life time.

*Therapist: "View the whole scene in slow motion and tell me. As all this is happening, what are you doing?"*

*Client: "I am trying to run out of the room, but the floor is shaking and almost broken. I feel trapped. The ceiling is falling on me and I can't run."*

*Therapist: "As this is happening, what are you feeling?"*

*Client: "I am feeling so scared; I am confused what should I do? Oh no... no, no, no, no... the ceiling has fallen on me. Holy shit! I am feeling so heavy."*

*After a brief pause, the client sighed and remarked quietly: "I am stuck."*

*Therapist: "As the ceiling has fallen on you and you are feeling stuck, what are you thinking?"*

*Client: "I am feeling, what will happen now? How long will I remain stuck here? I feel I will die now?"*

*Therapist: "Did you die?"*

*Client: "Yes, I died."*

*Therapist: "That life is now over and now, tell me, when did that past life get triggered in your current life."*

*Client: "2 months ago."*

*Therapist: "What happened 2 months ago, when you experienced similar emotions and thoughts?"*

*Client: "Yeah! I was thinking of investing in a new commercial space."*

*Therapist: "What were you thinking and feeling while taking the decision?"*

*Client: "I was feeling very apprehensive, as it was a new project. I was anxious to make the decision. I was constantly thinking, whether that mall project will be successful or a flop? And, what if my money gets stuck? And my father was pressuring me to invest in that project, as it was his friend's project."*

*Therapist: "So what did that make you feel?"*

*Client: "I was feeling so stuck, so confused, so helpless... I did not know what to do."*

Client felt exactly same emotions in the present life, as he felt in his past life.

*Therapist: "Try to recall that you started experiencing loose motions, stomach cramps and nausea, during or after that episode?"*

*Client: "Yes, I remember now, that my loose motions began the day I invested in that project."*

*Therapist: "Do you now realize how your father's pressure and stress led to stomach problems?*

*Client: "Yes."*

*Therapist: "Do you feel the stomach cramps or dizziness now?"*

*Client: "No, I am fine now. I feel so relieved. Thank you!"*

*After self-realization and healing, the lovely session ended.*

**Therapist Conclusion:**

The therapy session was very clear and self-explanatory. It was when Manish was forced by his father to invest in a project that he felt scared and helpless. He was confused and felt trapped in a constant loop of overthinking that triggered his past life in which he died feeling similar emotions and thoughts. He was stuck under the ceiling, in that past life and could not move, so it was a similar situation in his present life, when his father was forcing him to invest in the project and he was scared and confused about its performance in the future. But because of his father's pressures, he felt trapped and helpless. Consequently, he suffered from loose motions and stomach cramps. Through the beautiful therapy session, Manish was released from extreme fear of the unknown and his past intense emotions that adversely affected his health. After a week, Manish called and told me that he was absolutely fine and his physical symptoms did not relapse, even after he stopped his medication.

Guidance: If you are experiencing stomach problems, then it is your mind that is causing you to suffer. Instead of suppressing your problem by taking medications, it is advisable to clear your mind and deal with the real root cause of your issue. You can prevent the problem from recurring.

**Healing Stomach Ailments:**

**Transpersonal Regression Therapy:** Regression Therapies are the fastest way to heal stomach issues because they work on your subconscious mind and lead to deep healing. Since stomach is the first part of your body that gets affected due to overthinking or negative thought processes, it is essential to heal your mind. When you heal your mind and identify the core issue then your stomach problems automatically get healed.

**Think Positive**: In order to keep your stomach clean, keep your thoughts positive. Do not clog your mind with negative thoughts. Clogged mind will lead to a clogged stomach. Consequently, a clogged stomach will lead to stomach problems.

**Avoid Overthinking**: While taking any major decisions, remember, to only analyse the pros and cons. In the light of your present knowledge, take a wise decision. Once the decision is taken then, don't think about it again. Try to implement your ideas and keep moving ahead with confidence. If you get any obstacles and your heart feels like you need to amend your decision, then don't analyse it again, simply change your decision. You have to understand that you need to flow with the universe not against it. Be aware of universal synchronicities. Don't dwell into overthinking or negative self-sabotaging statements.

Overthinking will only confuse you. So, remember, once you take the decision, don't give it a second thought. Only if there are any blockages in your path, then immediately change your path. This will help to make right decisions without any confusions, and this will also help you gain confidence in yourself. But for some reason, if it is not possible to change the decision then that means it's destiny. Don't try to change your decision or think negatively at that moment. Remember, you have a choice of freewill, but destiny will take its course, you cannot change it. Keep moving with faith. Initially, you may feel uncomfortable to walk the unknown path, but if it's destined, then it implies that it is a part of your life plan, and you are closer to your sole purpose. Enjoy your journey rather than feeling stressed about it. Believe that everything happens for a reason, and everything happens for your highest good.

**Avoid Self-Criticism and Guilt**: The decision you take is your choice of freewill, but the result is not in your hands. So, once you make your decision and everything begins to flow without any obstacles then just feel satisfied with your decision. Maintain peace with yourself, that you have chosen the best in your capacity. Remember, you can only make decisions in the light of the best possible knowledge. You have control over the decision, not over the result. The consequence of your decision is already predestined, it is not your mistake. After all, it is your destiny.

**Let go of Past**: It is necessary to release your past memories. To heal your stomach issues, it is important to heal your mind. Free yourself from the traumatic memories that have chained you to your past. Forgive everyone with understanding. Try to focus on your past and analyse how did it bring out the best version of you, today? Just recall how it was beneficial to you. focus on the strengths that you developed after that episode. Remember to focus only on the positive attributes. This will help you to attain peace and satisfaction.

## CHAKRAS

**Solar Plexus Chakra**: Solar plexus chakra is the chakra of control. So, whenever there is loss of control in your life, then the solar plexus chakra is imbalanced. Stomach belongs to a part of your solar plexus chakra, so whenever there are negative thoughts in your mind, then your stomach gets upset as your solar plexus chakra gets either partially blocked or completely blocked. As you read about the chakras in our body. You will be able to learn more about how to heal your stomach related problems and diseases.

**Heart Chakra and Sacral Chakra:** Along with the solar plexus chakra, your heart chakra and the sacral Chakra also get blocked whenever your mind gets clogged with negative thoughts and emotions. Whenever you start feeling guilty or helpless due to some people or events in life, then initially your heart chakra starts getting imbalanced or partially blocked. Consequently, you feel loss of control over your own mind and body due to which your solar plexus chakra gets imbalanced. You begin to feel very low. You experience a state of feeling intense emotions like guilt, helplessness, self-criticism and anger. Ultimately, the blanket of these dark emotions takes over your control completely. Have you ever seen a beautiful sky suddenly getting covered with the mist of dark clouds? Negative thought processes clog your mind, just like that mist of dark clouds. You start feeling unhappy and unsatisfied in life, as a result your sacral chakra also gets blocked.

**Emotion Management Technique:** You can chant 'guilt' or 'helpless' to surface the physical sensations, and then follow the EMT steps mentioned under the "Emotion Management Techniques" section in the "Healing" Chapter of the book.

**Positive Affirmations**

**Constipation or Stomach Ulcer:**

*"I release with understanding."*

*"I forgive with awareness."*

*"I release with love."*

*"I love and accept myself as I am."*

*"I forgive myself."*

**Acidity, Gas, or Abdominal Pains or Loose Motions:**

*"I digest all the ideas with easily."*

*"I assimilate everything around me with understanding."*

*"I have faith in the divine process."*

*"I love accept myself as I am."*

*"I forgive myself."*

Meditation to release yourself and bring peace of mind. You can refer to the meditation section under the healing chapter of the book.

## LIVER:
## "I feel angry over people and the entire authoritative system."

### Do you feel extremely annoyed over the Authoritative system?

Majority of the cases who experienced fatty liver, abnormal levels of SGPT or SGOT and liver cirrhosis displayed a common pattern of intolerance towards injustice and corrupted authoritative systems. They felt helpless and frustrated due to the prevailing unjust conditions, but were unable to change them. They kept supressing their emotions which was the major cause of their Liver problems. If you are suffering from liver problems, then you may be having low tolerance towards injustice. These emotions get intensified when you perceive similar unjust behaviour of people towards you or other people as a result you suffer with fatty liver and also continue to attract repeated patterns of misunderstanding and disputes with the people around you. Thus, it is your beliefs formed due to your past experiences and the repressed emotions that lead to recurring health problems and stressful relationships.

### Do you wonder why you cannot say "No" to your parents and loved ones?

Through my case studies, it was also evident that if you are suffering from fatty liver then you may be carrying subconscious anger over parents and tolerating certain stubborn and rude behaviour of your family members. You continue to take care of your loved ones, ignoring your own needs, just worrying about everyone around you and wishing for the best for all of them, but all in vain as they never value your emotions. You continue to suppress your rage and frustrations. This discontent and frustration is then directed towards your workplace, at your employees or coworkers, resulting in more misunderstandings or disputes. It impacts not only your relationships with others, but it may also lead to financial struggles because stress causes you to lose focus at work, and repeated workplace squabbles can lead to job loss or financial incompetence.

Most of my clients who were suffering from liver problems were the most obedient children to their parents. You must be wondering how being obedient or taking too much care of parents and your loved ones could damage your liver? Right? So, let's understand this through the following case study.

**Case Study**

Amreek, who was 45 years old, was suffering from very high levels of SGPT and SGOT, so he wanted to heal the root cause of these abnormal levels of liver cells. He was very scared as the doctors warned him that his liver was in danger. So, the Regression therapy session was conducted. It was a beautiful session that will help you to realise how during your childhood you innocently form certain beliefs that influence your later life.

**Therapy Session:**

Amreek was induced a deep trance state and the therapy session commenced.

*Therapist: "How does the very thought of liver might get damaged, makes you feel?"*

*Client: "I feel I should do my best to take care and not let that happen."*

*Therapist: "Are you doing your best?"*

*Client: "Yes."*

*Therapist: "Then, what makes you so worried?"*

*Client: "I feel apprehensive, what if I am not able to take care of it properly? then my liver will get damaged."*

*Therapist: "Feel this apprehensiveness and let me know, where in your body, do you feel it?"*

*Client: "I am feeling pain in my abdomen."*

*Therapist: "How does it make you feel?"*

*Client: "I am feeling scared and helpless."*

*Therapist: "Invite that age of you who is feeling so scared and helpless. How old are you?"*

*Client: "I am 7 years old."*

*Therapist: "Go back in time to your age of 7 and recall why you are feeling so scared and helpless?"*

*Client: "I am standing outside the room of my parents, I heard my mother telling my father that he should be strict with me."*

*Therapist: "Why do you think that your mother said this to your father?"*

*Client: "I was very naughty, so I feel she warned my father to be strict with me."*

*Therapist: "How did this make you feel?"*

*Client: "My father was very aggressive and used to scold me a lot, so I got very frightened that he would not spare me, if I commit any mistake."*

*Therapist: "Why did you feel that he would not spare you?"*

*Client: "Because he was so impulsive, he used to hit my mother. So, I felt that if I would not obey him, then he would hit me also."*

*Therapist: "So, what did you decide?"*

*Client: "I decided to always obey him and never give him any reasons to hit me."*

*Therapist: "How did you do this?"*

*Client: "I became a very obedient son, I always listened to him and decided to never say "No" to him."*

*Therapist: "So, you did whatever he asked you?"*

*Client: "Yes, even if I didn't wish to, I used to fulfil his wishes."*

*Therapist: "How did that make you feel?"*

*Client: "I felt very helpless, sometimes angry."*

*Therapist: "How did this affect your later life?"*

*Client: "My whole life revolved around my parents."*

*Therapist: "How did this make you feel?"*

*Client: "I almost forgot my own needs; even my wife sometimes quarrelled with me for always being a Yes Man to my father. At times we all felt that he was illogical and unreasonable. But I could never dare to oppose him."*

*Therapist: "Is your father dominating today also?"*

*Client: "Yes, he is but we share a very good bond and I'm not scared of him."*

*After the beautiful self-realization, the 7 years old inner child was healed and integrated with the adult Amreek.*

*Therapist: "Any pains in your abdominal pain?"*

*Client: "No, it's fine now."*

*The session then ended.*

**Therapist Conclusion:**

Through the trance session, it was concluded that it was the 7 years old inner child who was frightened of his impulsive father and thus, he concluded that he had to always obey him, otherwise he would hit him also like his mother. The child decided to never oppose his father, so he continued to obey his unreasonable demands. The adult Amreek felt angry and helpless and was suffering because the seven years old inner child was extremely horrified by his father's impulsive behaviour. Although the adult Amreek consciously was aware that his father had changed a lot and he shared a very loving relationship with him now, but 7 years old inner child remained stuck in the past memories and beliefs.

Being obedient or taking too much care of your parents doesn't lead to liver problems, it is your fear, helplessness and anger towards parents that leads to liver damage. If you develop subconscious fear and anger towards your parents during your childhood, then this anger and helplessness keeps growing in your later life. These unhealed emotions continue to resurface during similar traumatic episodes with your loved ones, which in turn, affects your health.

Liver never starts damaging instantly. When there is a lot of suppressed anger and helplessness, then it leads to excess production of bile juice. Bile juice is required in a particular quantity to digest the food particles. But if it is secreted in excess, then it affects your stomach. Consequently, it leads to physical symptoms like burning sensations, acidity, gas, constipation, etc.

My purpose in writing this book is to make you understand that whenever your stomach is upset, then at that level only you should understand and treat your subconsciously stored unhealed emotions as it could be dangerous to other organs.

**Healing Liver Issues:**

**Regression therapy** is the best method to heal the inner child and liberate the adult you who feels shackled in chains of the past. Hypnotherapy and other transpersonal therapies are the most effective techniques that lead to deep introspection and self-realization, which in turn helps in better understanding and faster recovery of not only health problems but also relationship issues.

**Anger Control**: You can heal your liver problems by controlling your anger. Most of my clients stated that they don't feel angry, in fact they share very good bonding with their parents and loved ones. And that is the reason, exactly, why I am sharing this example with you. When there is an argument with your loved one or you feel that they are behaving irrationally with you then just keep quiet for some time. In that quiet moment, think, "What did I do?" You may not have done anything at that moment, but maybe your loved ones are carrying a memory of your past behaviour. Change the way you respond. Give them time. Express your sentiments later to them. Then you will be surprised to see their response. When you change your perspective and view things with the other person's point of view, then your bond with them will become stronger than before.

Do you wonder, that sometimes, after your impulsive reaction, you feel guilty that you overreacted? This is a consequence of a repressed childhood anger, which you may or may not be aware of. You are the most obedient child of your parents. You sometimes have to listen to them despite your heart's protests. You never express your actual emotions to them as a result, you suppress your deepest emotions. This can also adversely affect your health. Don't suppress your sentiments. Express your emotions clearly to your loved ones. There is a difference between respect and fear. It is essential for you to understand that respecting your elders is the key to buildings healthy relationships with your parents. Respect your parents and do everything for them out of love rather than fear. When you deal with every situation with love and acceptance, then you will never develop repressed emotions or bitterness, subconsciously. Healthy mind will in turn result in a healthy life and strong relationship bonds.

**Self-love:** Love and accept yourself as you are. Take care of yourself along with the same love and compassion for your loved ones. Listen to your heart. Follow your inner voice. Remember, it is okay to say "No" if you don't feel right. Stop feeling guilty. Liberate yourself from all the burdens of proving yourself as the best child. Your parents will love you despite your actions. Avoid sabotaging yourself. Guilt leads to stomach problems. So, it is very important to stop criticizing yourself. You can also follow the healing methods mentioned for curing your stomach issues in the abdominal issues chapter.

**Chakras:** Liver is also a part of solar plexus chakra. So, your solar plexus chakra is imbalanced. In fact, your heart chakra as well as your sacral chakra also gets blocked, when your solar plexus chakra is imbalanced. You have to take charge of your own life. Forgive everyone around you who had wounded your heart. Understand other persons perspectives and analyse their versions in every past traumatic situation with them. This will help you to forgive them easily. You can refer to the chakra chapter to learn about the balancing and activation of your chakras.

**Emotion Management Technique:** You can chant 'anger' to surface the physical sensations and then follow the EMT steps mentioned under the "Emotion Management Techniques" section under the "Healing" Chapter of the book.

## KIDNEY:
## "I feel angry over parents and siblings."

**Do you feel that your siblings or your parents or other loved ones didn't treat you the way you deserved?**

You may suffer with kidney stones or kidney problems when you feel that you were available to your loved ones during their thick and thin, but they never reciprocated in the same manner. You loved them wholeheartedly, ignored yourself and your family for them but they always blamed you. You were always a happy and fulfilled and satisfied soul, but their behaviour forced you towards negative thinking and criticism. You wonder that you were such a positive person, but they made you feel small and guilty over petty issues. They badly impacted you to the point where you started feeling annoyed about everything in life.

Majority of the people who suffer with kidney issues have a habit of cribbing. It is their criticizing nature that causes damage to their kidneys. The stored anger and resentment can lead to kidney stones too.

**Case Study**

Vikas, who was 47 years old complained of kidney stones. He got the Lasik treatment done and got rid of the stones, but later his right kidney began to deteriorate. He was completely confused and worried as the doctors were clueless and failed to understand the reason for the organ deterioration. He was mentally frazzled, he couldn't concentrate at work, and as a result, he was facing financial challenges. He began to feel agitated and frustrated, which led to disagreements with his spouse and disillusionment.

He consulted me to cope with his depression but as he delved deep into his mysterious subconscious mind, confusions receded into the background, reflecting the true source of his prolonged struggle. It was a very beautiful eye opening and heart touching therapy session.

In the trance state, it was revealed that when Vikas was 7 years old, his father told him that he was the eldest son and thus, it was his responsibility to take care of his siblings. He had one sister and one brother. The 7 years old Vikas subconsciously developed a false pride of being the eldest and a superiority complex. Consciously, he was only obeying his father's decision to take care of his siblings but unconsciously, he began to dominate and control his siblings. He felt that he was the eldest and his father had given him the authority to mend them and make them good human beings. His siblings were terrified by his behaviour. They subconsciously developed a lot of rage over him. Until they were young, they quietly obeyed him, but when they grew old, they resorted to a lot of disagreements and conflicts. Consciously, they respected him but stored a lot of resentment in their heart. Gradually, they distanced themselves from him.

He added that in spite of separation, he never turned his back over them. He was always available to his sister and brother in times of their crisis, but they always took advantage of his love. He felt that they were very selfish and only remembered him when they needed him.

Through the therapy session, it was discovered that it was the 7 years old inner child of Vikas who was stuck with the responsibility syndrome due to which the adult Vikas was suffering. Adult Vikas could not accept his sibling's behaviour, but still felt chained to them because it was the 7 years old inner child who felt obligated by his father's assertions. Adult Vikas failed to understand the reason why he felt so responsible for the well-being of his siblings though they didn't deserve his love and care. He mentioned that he tried to control his emotions and detach from them. He tried to recall their inappropriate past behaviours with him to find some reasonable reasons to keep away from them, but then he felt extremely guilty for not being there for them throughout their turmoil period, and helpless showed up and later felt even more guilty when they turned their back over him.

Through the beautiful contemplation in the trance state, the 7 years old inner child was liberated from the shackles of the obligation bestowed upon him by his father, and the adult Vikas was freed from all the conflicting emotions that had caused emotional damage. Vikas got answers to all his questions like “Why me?” It was a very deep and satisfying session which concluded with beautiful self-realization. Vikas was out of the victim mode and blame game. However, Vikas still had to undergo the kidney transplant. But after the healing of the inner child and his renewed perspectives, it is possible that his new kidney will not be in danger now.

Transplantation of the organ is possible, but if the underlying cause of the deterioration of your organ remains unresolved, the new organ that is transplanted may be at risk of damage again. Thus, rather than escaping the triggered unhealed emotions, it is vital to identify and treat the root causes of your problem. Heal the primary cause of your issues rather than suppressing them.

**Healing Kindly Ailments:**

**Regression Therapy:** Regression Therapy sessions and inner child work are the most effective methods to heal the root cause of the organ damage or stone related issues. Treating the deep-rooted unhealed emotions and releasing the negative postulates or oaths taken during childhood liberates the adult from further damage both emotionally as well as physically. Inner child work and Regression Therapies assist in self-realization that result in cathartic moments which help in deep healing. Moreover, it provides answers to their individual questions, "Why me?" Psychological counselling is not much effective in such cases as they are done at the conscious mind level. Hypnotherapy and regression therapies aid in achieving deep insights and self-realization which help to achieve better understanding of the real problem.

**Chakras:** In case of kidney problems, your heart chakra, solar plexus chakra and the sacral chakra are imbalanced. Major emotions that need to be healed are guilt, helplessness and criticism. You have to take charge of your own emotions. Avoid becoming agitated over insignificant issues. Maintain calmness at all times.

**Emotion Management Technique:** You can chant 'guilt' or 'helpless' to surface the physical sensations and then follow the EMT steps mentioned under the "Emotion Management Techniques" section under the "Healing" Chapter of the book.

Change your perspective. If there had been wrong people in the past, then that doesn't mean that the entire world is wrong. You can trust other people. Be receptive, don't close yourself in the cocoon of self-limited beliefs. Open your heart towards your loved ones and do everything with zero expectations. It will never lead to any guilt, helplessness or resentment. They are your karmic relations. They are meant to be there in your life, so accept them as they are. Yes, you can choose to be there for them or not, it's your decision. Make your choices clearly but avoid criticism. It's not worth it, it will only damage you internally.

Your health is important. For good health, a positive mindset is the key. Increase your will power to live. Be grateful to all the people who made you so strong. Focus on your past weaknesses which no longer exist in your system. Your karmic teachers have changed you tremendously and you could shine with flying colours, acknowledge that shift in you.

Focus on all the positive events, people and possessions that you have. This will help you to increase happiness within you naturally. Try it!

Meditation for forgiveness in the "Healing" chapter of the book can be done to release yourself from the suppressed traumatic past memories and heal your wounded heart.

# Chapter 11
# ANAL PAINS AND DISEASES

**Do you have a habit of taking stubborn oaths?**

For instance, if someone has caused you pain, then you consciously formulate certain stubborn rules for yourselves in regard to that individual and abide by them, at all costs. You forgive them consciously, if they want to resolve the matter but deep within your heart, you continue to carry the wound for your entire life.

## FISSURES AND PILES:

***"I feel stuck in my life."***

Are your finances stuck? When you are encountering stress due to finances or when your horrified past keeps plaguing your present, then it affects not only your stomach, but it can lead to anal problems as well. Issues like piles, fissures and other anal problems never begin suddenly, it is a consequence of persistent constipation. As mentioned previously, constipation occurs when you are facing financial instabilities or stuck in your past, refusing to forgive people who hurt or betrayed you. This results in sensations in your anal or rectum areas: itching, burning, rashes or diseases like fissures, piles, etc. can be experienced. To illustrate, let's understand this through the following case of Romil.

**Case Study**

Romil, who was 38 years old, was suffering from anal issues and severe constipation as well as blood in her stool. She wanted to avoid surgery and that is why she wanted to seek Regression Therapy to heal the root cause. She was informed by the doctors that she was suffering because of her food habits. She was confused because she was on a very healthy diet, but still her problem persisted. Through the astounding therapy session, the dust of her confusion settled, and she gained clarity in certain dark episodes of her life which were the actual root cause of her consistent pain and bleeding. This beautiful session will make you realize that sometimes you feel that you have forgotten your past and forgiven the people who hurt you but deep within you the scars of the old wounds keep triggering in your current reality, unconsciously.

**Therapy Session:**

After a deep hypnotic state was induced, the therapy session began.

*Therapist: "When you see the blood in your stool, then how does it make you feel?"*

*Client: "Oh, I feel terrified. It's disgusting and frustrating."*

*Therapist: "Just get all the impressions of the thoughts which come to your mind at that moment."*

*Client: "I feel very helpless and tired. I keep wondering when will it stop? I have consulted so many dietitians. I have amended my diet plans. I can't even eat my favourite dishes. I've taken all the necessary steps to heal it, but all in vain; I'm perplexed. Sometimes I wonder what am I missing?"*

*Therapist: "Reason for this blood in your stool is standing outside the door. Open the door and let me know, who is it? First thought, first impression."*

*Client: "It's my elder sister, Tarang."*

*Therapist: "What age has Tarang entered into the room?"*

*Client: "37 years."*

*Therapist: "How old were you when she was 37 years old?"*

*Client: "I was 32 years old."*

*Therapist: "What happened when you were 32 years old that made you feel so frustrated and confused, as if you were missing something?"*

*Client started feeling acute lower abdominal pain.*

*Therapist: "What is happening?"*

*Client cried: "I'm feeling a lot of pain below my stomach."*

*Suddenly, Romil yelled loudly: "She cheated on me. She slept with my husband. She was going through a difficult married life, so I tried to help her and brought her to my house for a few days. I did not have a clue of what was going on... Oh! I'm so foolish, I did even realize that they were sleeping under my nose..."*

*Tears rolled down her beautiful eyes.*

*Therapist: "What did you do?"*

*The sobbing client wiped her tears away and relentlessly: "I chucked both of them out of my house."*

*Client: "I have applied for a divorce."*

*Therapist: "Did you confront your husband?"*

*Client: "Yes, I did confront him, and he tried to convince me of his shameful act, but I didn't listen to him. Instead, I threw all his stuff out of my house in the middle of the night."*

*Therapist: "After that episode, did your husband try to reconcile?"*

*Client: "Yes, many times he's tried to call me. He was feeling guilty, but I could not forgive him."*

*Therapist: "Are you both legally divorced now?"*

*Client: "Yes, we are divorced and I am married to a very kind-hearted and trustworthy person now. In fact, I believe that everything happens for a reason and feel very calm now. However, that incident still haunts me at times. But I am grateful to my ex-husband, because if he hadn't cheated on me, I would never have met this beautiful Angel."*

*Therapist: "Now as you understand that everything had happened for a reason, are you ready to forgive your ex-husband?"*

*Client: "Yes, I have already forgiven him now."*

*After the intense catharsis and self-realization, the 32 years old inner child of Romil was healed and physical sensations were checked.*

*Therapist: "Do you feel any physical discomfort, now?"*

*Client: "No, I am absolutely fine."*

*Although a lengthy, but extremely insightful session ended.*

**Therapist Conclusion:**

Through the therapy session, it was concluded that the 38 years old Romil had moved on and forgiven her ex-husband for cheating on her, but the 32 years old inner child Romil was stuck with the past memory, feeling furious over her ex-husband. That event traumatized her, and she could not bear the feeling of rejection. Consequently, she decided to move on and release herself from the horrified memory. Consciously, she tried to forgive him as she married another person, who was better than him, but since she was deeply hurt by her ex-husband, she could not forgive him subconsciously. Simmering deep within was rage towards her ex-husband which led to severe pain in her anus and led to bleeding in her stool. After just one therapy session, Romil testified that the blood in her stool had stopped. She felt delighted as she could now eat her favourite food without fear. She also mentioned that she was feeling stuck in her previous job for past 2 years and had been struggling for a raise in salary, after the session she could see a tremendous movement in her life. She got promotion and her relationship with other people also improved.

As mentioned in the first chapter of this book, if your mind is stuck in any one area of your life, whether it's your relationship, health, or finances, you'll feel stuck in all the other spheres of your life. For instance, when your mind becomes stuck and it makes you feel helpless, then you feel the same helplessness in every other aspect of your life. To break the cycle of feeling helpless and stuck, you must stop resisting life's flow. When you begin to move with awareness and a happy attitude, you will notice a shift in yourself and in every sphere of your life. Try it!

**Healing Anal Issues:**

**Transpersonal Regression Therapy:** Transpersonal Regression Therapies as well as seeking counselling are very effective ways to heal anal and rectal problems as they can help you to achieve the cathartic moments and self-realization. However, Regression therapies heal at the subconscious level and impart insight to the conscious mind. Inevitably Transpersonal Regression therapies is the most potent approach to release you from your damaged past. In case you are suffering due to financial imbalances then Regression therapies help you to identify the primary root cause that are causing financial obstacles in your life. You will be able to achieve outstanding outcomes in just one therapy session.

**Forgiveness and Gratitude:** It is important to practice forgiveness and gratitude. Let go of your past and keep thanking people who hurt you. Positive thinking brings clarity. When you look at the entire episode as a spectator with a pleasant attitude, everything appears to be transparent as a mirror. Just like in the case of Romil, betrayal turned into blessings. Thus, it is important to overview the whole episode and focus on the benefits that you gained. Don't see yourself as the victim. Come out of the blame and focus on the blessings that you have in the present.

**Chakras:** Root chakra and sacral chakra are either partially blocked or completely blocked. To heal the anal problems, you have to balance your root chakra and the sacral chakra. Else it can lead to financial instability and a lot of anxiety issues. Kindly refer to the Chakra section to heal and activate them.

**Emotion Management Technique:** You can chant 'anger' or 'helpless' to surface the physical sensations, and then follow the EMT steps mentioned under the "Emotion Management Techniques" section under the "Healing" chapter of the book.

Meditation for forgiveness can be done in the book's "Healing" Chapter to liberate yourself from buried painful traumatic past memories and event. This will assist you to naturally heal your subconscious mind and heal you to the core.

# Chapter 12
# JOINT PAINS, SWELLINGS AND STIFFNESS

**Do you wonder why you become very rigid in making decisions for yourself or your family? Do you feel irritated and angry when somebody tries to impose their decisions on you or tries to change your perspective? Do you feel that you become very defensive, towards yourself and your loved ones during arguments?**

If yes, then you may be suffering from joint pains or stiffness in your neck, shoulders, back, hands, elbows, fingers, knees or ankle or arthritis. After extensive research on all the clients who reported stiffness in different parts of their body, it was observed that people who were very stubborn in nature, suffered from stiffness or arthritis.

*Do you feel that you cannot tolerate injustice? Do you feel that you have to stand up for yourself and defend? Are you one of those who feels very restless till you prove your point?*

Then, please be aware of your thought processes and actions, because they can lead you to experience severe joint pains, stiffness or swellings. However, it depends which part of your body or joint starts hurting you first, as different emotions affect different parts of your body. As you read further, you will understand the real cause of your pain in different parts of your body.

## ARTHRITIS:
## "Please don't tell me what to do?"

It is a medical condition which leads to joint pains and swellings in neck, shoulders, hands, elbows, wrists, fingers, knees, etc.

**Do you wonder why you get stuck in a loop till you get a logical reason for your question?**

If yes, then it is this rigidity in your thought process that leads to stiffness in your physical body. You are one of those who doesn't like to run away from your problems or discussions. You like to deal with your issues and solve them. The good quality in you is that you are very analytical and convince people with your logical reasoning, but sometimes you do not want to understand another person's perspective. You try to defend yourself as much as you can, but when the argument is with your loved ones then all your defences break down. You try to compromise for their sake. You surrender just to finish the conversation, to maintain peace in the environment or in your relationships, but subconsciously your mind is stuck with the thought that you are the only one who, ultimately has to always compromise. You always feel like a victim. You feel angry and helpless, but keep quiet and that is the reason you start developing body pains and stiffness.

Pain and swelling are also associated with guilt and storing past, old wounds and hurts (as mentioned in the Abdominal Pains Chapter). Majority of my clients, who suffered from joint pains and swellings, displayed a pattern of always feeling guilty. Just try to recall: **Do you have a tendency to feel guilty after having an argument with your loved ones? Do you sometimes wonder that you overreact?** Yes, with your loved ones all your defence mechanisms break down and you feel guilty for your actions and words. This is the actual reason, why you develop pains and swellings in your body. You will gain more clarity on this concept as you read further.

## NECK PAIN:
## "I cannot tolerate domination."

Do you wonder why, although you are very open to suggestions but become extremely agitated when some tries to impose their decisions on you? This happens because consciously, you feel that you are open to advices from others but you have very strong opinions and beliefs, therefore you don't like when people tell you what to do and how to do things?

Have you ever noticed a bull? The bull looks only in one direction, even though it may move in all the directions. My case studies revealed that most of my clients who complained of neck pains or stiffness were very stubborn in nature and resisted change. They preferred to suffer rather than change.

Do you feel that you have a very stern or rigid thought process? If yes, then you must be suffering from stiffness or pains. You hold very strong a belief system and you just don't like to change your perspective unless you get a logical answer, as mentioned earlier. This rigidity in your thought process is the root cause for your neck pain. Let's understand this with the following case study.

### Case Study

A client consulted me for her severe neck pain and arthritis. Before the session, she completely denied that she was stubborn. Rather, she mentioned that she was a very adjusting and compromising person in her whole family. So, the Regression Therapy session was conducted which was a phenomenal and awestruck experience that left her speechless.

### Therapy Session:

After a deep hypnotic state was induced, therapy session began.

*Therapist: "Are you feeling neck pain right now?"*

*Client: "Yes."*

*Therapist: "Breathe into this pain and feel it growing."*

*Client started scratching her arms and face.*

*Therapist: "What is happening?"*

*Client: "I am feeling itching and pain in my right arm."*

*Therapist: "How does that make you feel?"*

*Client: "I am feeling very irritated. I don't understand, what's going on? I feel confused, will my pains be healed, ever?"*

*Therapist: "As you are feeling irritated and confused, it reminds you of?"*

*Client: "My grandfather."*

*Therapist: "How old are you feeling irritated with your grandfather?"*

*Client: "I am 4 years old."*

*Therapist: "Why are you feeling irritated with your grandfather?"*

*Client: "He is scolding my mother."*

*Therapist: " When he is scolding your mother, then what are you feeling?"*

*Client: "I am feeling very angry and confused. I don't understand why is he always scolding my mother?"*

*Therapist: "What did you do?"*

*Client: "I started throwing things down from the table, and ran to stop him."*

*Therapist: "Did he stop, then?"*

*Client: "Yes, when I threw things then he stopped for a moment, but then again, he continued scolding my mother. So, I came back and threw more things and again ran."*

*Therapist: "Then what happened?"*

*Client: "Then he ran after me and scolded me."*

*Therapist: "What did you feel?"*

*Client: "I felt scared and anxious, but I decided that I will not stop until he stopped scolding my mother."*

*Therapist: "Then, did he stop?"*

*Client: "Yes."*

*Therapist: "How did this incident impact your actions, later as you grew older?"*

*Client: "I feel I could not tolerate injustice. These authority figures irritated me. I felt a need to stand up for myself and people who were weak."*

*Therapist: "So do you feel that you have a very strong opinion about authority figures?"*

*Client: "Yes, I just can't tolerate any domination."*

*Therapist: "Do you feel that you are stubborn and have rigid point of views."*

*Client: "Yes, definitely. I don't listen to people who try to impose their decisions on me. In fact, I continue to argue, till they understand my point."*

*Client cried loudly: "Oh my God, I am feeling a lot of pain in my neck."*

*Therapist: "What does this pain remind you of?"*

*Client: "It reminds me of my grandfather and all the other dominating people in my life, especially men. All of them are a pain in my neck."*

*The 4 years old inner child feeling irritated and confused was healed, and self-realization was brought to the client.*

*Therapist: "Now, do you understand that this rigid thought process and stubbornness of the 4 years old child was the root cause of your neck pain and arthritis?"*

*Client: "Yes."*

*Therapist: "Do you feel any pain now?"*

*Client: "No, I don't feel any pain now."*

*After the beautiful revelation and self-realization, healing was done and the therapy session ended.*

**Therapist Conclusion:**

After the healing session, the client told me that she was a divorcee. She stated that after the session, she realized that it was the inner child who was stuck in the past, feeling scared of her grandfather. It was the child who had developed anger towards the authority figures, especially towards men. As a result of this, her adult self, faced issues in her marriage. She also accepted that she was scared of changing her perspectives. She used to feel agitated if somebody tried to control her or impose their decisions on her. She accepted and acknowledged unconscious parts of her personality which helped her to heal at a deeper level. She felt better after the session. She was made aware that her rigidity and resistance were causing her stiffness and pain in her neck, so it was her responsibility to take care of her attitudes and perspectives in future.

**Healing Neck Pains:**

**Deep Introspection:** Whenever you are suffering from neck pain, then find a quiet space and sit down in solace for some time. Just focus on your breath and ask yourself, "Who is the pain in your neck? Is it worth taking pain for that person?" Release yourself from the energies of that person by forgiving him/her. And if you find it difficult to do so or you still suffer with pain then take Regression therapy. Transpersonal Regression therapy is the best way to heal the inner children. Other pain-relieving treatments include Physiotherapy, Acupuncture, and Acupressure.

**Listen to Others' Perspectives:** Try to understand another person's perspective. When you try to understand another person's perspective, then it leads to healthy discussions rather than arguments. Listen to people's advice but follow your heart. Do as you wish.

**Positive Thinking:** It is important to change your thought process and stop being defensive while talking to other people. Try to learn from other people.

**Accept Change:** Change is the most permanent phenomenon on Earth. Don't take change as a challenge. Consider it as an opportunity to grow. There is a difference between compromise and acceptance. Compromise means that you are accepting the situation helplessly not with proper understanding. Therefore, you may suffer from stiffness in your body. If you accept the situation happily, then you will never develop stiffness in your body.

**Empathy:** Yes, self-love is very important. You should love yourself, but you should also take care of the other people with the same love and compassion. When you understand other person's perspectives and pains, then you get a better understanding of the situation. It becomes easier for you to forgive.

**Gratitude and Forgiveness:** Thank everyone around you, especially your enemies, as they help you to focus on your weaknesses and change your weakness into strengths. They help you to become the best version out of you. For instance, the majority of my clients claimed that their karmic teachers assisted them in gaining confidence. Many of them said they were introverts and shy during their childhood, but their karmic teachers' interference encouraged them to stand up for themselves, and as a result, they became very expressive.

**Chakras:** Third eye chakra, throat chakra and heart chakra are imbalanced, so learn to balance and activate them. Kindly refer to the Chakra healing section.

**Affirmations:**

*"I feel safe to change."*

*"I feel safe to listen to others."*

*"I feel safe to communicate."*

*"I feel safe to express myself."*

## SHOULDER PAIN:
## "I am overburdened with responsibilities."

**Do you wonder why you are always overburdened with responsibilities?**

Majority of my clients who reported shoulder pains displayed a pattern of being overburdened by the responsibilities of their loved ones. If you are suffering from pains or heaviness in your shoulders then you are doing more than your capacity. You are subconsciously feeling helpless and burdened in your life which is the real cause of your shoulder discomfort. To illustrate, let's understand this with the following case study.

## Case Study

Mahim, who was 38 years old, complained of having severe cervical issues for the past 3 years, and therefore he wanted to take Regression Therapy to heal the root cause. It was an unexpected and very intense session as it unfolded. You'll be surprised to learn how, as a child, sometimes, you take oaths innocently, and then subconsciously or consciously, feel trapped with them for the rest of your life.

## Hypnotherapy Session:

*Therapist: "Breathe into your shoulder and feel your pain growing."*

*Client: "My pain is increasing."*

*Therapist: "How does that make you feel?"*

*Client: "I feel as if something heavy is put on my shoulders."*

*Therapist: "How is this heavy thing making you feel?"*

*Client: "I am feeling helpless and anxious."*

*Client started shaking. His legs and hands started shivering.*

*Therapist: "What are you feeling?"*

*Client: "I am feeling very scared and a severe pain in my ankle, as if it's twisted."*

*Therapist: "Go back to that moment when your ankle twisted, and you felt this helplessness very strongly."*

*Client cried out loudly: "I was 6 years old."*

*Therapist: "What happened, when you were 6 years old?"*

*Client: "My father died in front of me."*

*Therapist: "How did he die?"*

*Client: "I was holding the hand of my father, and we were walking on the street. I was trying to cross the road, but I did not look towards the left side and a fast moving truck was coming towards me. My father pushed me to the other end of the road to save me and he got crushed by the truck."*

*Therapist: "What happened next?"*

*Client: "My ankle twisted, and I could not save my father. I cried loudly for help, I felt very helpless. I could not move. My father tried to reach out to me, his hands and legs were shaking. I saw blood all around him, then I fainted."*

*Therapist: "When you gained consciousness, then where were you?"*

*Client: "I was in my room. I heard my mother crying loudly in the drawing room. I could not walk because my ankle was twisted, but I limped to the drawing room to see if my dad survived."*

*Therapist: "When you went to the drawing room, what did you see?"*

*Client: "I saw my father's dead body. I was shocked."*

*Therapist: "What did you feel?"*

*Client: "I cried a lot whenever I saw my mother depressed. I always blamed myself. I felt very guilty, but I was very weak, and also, very small. I could not do anything for my mother at that time."*

*Therapist: "You felt so weak, so small at that time, so what did you decide?"*

*Client: "I swore to take care of my mother when I grow up."*

*Therapist: "Did you take care of your mother when you grew big?"*

*Client started coughing.*

*Client: "Yes. I took care that she was never hurt. I always obeyed her. Today, also I do everything that she wants me to do, even if I don't wish to do. I never say 'No' to her."*

*Self-realization was brought to the client.*

*Therapist: "Do you understand how that decision is impacting your life today?"*

*Client: "Yes, now I understand."*

*6 years inner child of Mahim was healed and integrated, and then physical symptoms were checked.*

*Therapist: "Do you still feel the pain in your shoulders?"*

*Client: "No."*

*Therapist: "Do you still feel the pain in your left ankle?"*

*Client: "No, it is fine. Thank you."*

*The heart touching session ended after so much catharsis and deep contemplation.*

**Therapist Conclusion:**

Through the therapy session it was revealed that the 6 years old inner child of Mahim was stuck with the feelings of guilt, as his father died in the accident while saving him. The young child concluded that it was his responsibility to take care of the mother, as he blamed himself for his father's death. The coughing during the session very evidently proves that he could never express his own will to the mother. He silently continued to do as she wished. When you are not able to communicate your true feelings then your throat chakra gets affected. Your physical body keeps signalling you about the issues in your life. You just need to understand your own true self. Whenever you take burdens helplessly, then you develop shoulder problems. Cervical problems emerge in those who take on obligations helplessly and frequently feel guilty for not being able to do it flawlessly. After a month, Mahim testified that his shoulder pains were completely healed and he had stopped the cervical medicines also.

It is essential to be aware that you can take responsibilities of your loved ones but only in your capacity. You cannot change their destiny or reduce their sufferings. You should never take pledge or oaths over anything as you become stuck with them not only in your current life, but also in future lifetimes. Until you release yourself from the oaths, your suffering continues repeatedly. This may lead to guilt, helplessness and dissatisfaction due to which you subconsciously sabotage yourself. Consequently, it impacts not only your health, but also affects your relationships and finances.

**Healing Shoulder Problems:**

Transpersonal Regression Therapies is the best way to heal the inner children, stuck in the past memories or oaths. While other ways are:

**Self-understanding:** Taking responsibility is a noble job, but you have to remember that you can only do it in your capacity. Always take the responsibilities happily, and not with helplessness or guilt. Set boundaries for yourself and start saying ‘No’ when you feel tired. Enjoy doing things for others. Remember, that you are not God, you can commit mistakes. You don't have to feel guilty, for every small little thing. Work hard in your capacity and give your 100%. But remember that you don't have to be a perfectionist. Your intentions should be good. Take responsibilities out of your own free will and not because of others’ expectations. Pains and swellings develop only when you do the tasks helplessly.

**Chakras:** The throat chakra and heart chakra are imbalanced. To heal the shoulder problems. You have to activate and balance these chakras.

**Emotion Management Technique:** You can chant 'helpless' or 'fear' or 'anxiety' to surface the physical sensations, and then follow the EMT steps mentioned under the "Emotion Management Techniques" section under the "Healing" Chapter of the book.

**Affirmations:**

*"I take my responsibilities in my capacity."*

*"I take responsibilities happily."*

*"I love my work."*

*"I love to do things for others."*

*"I have faith in the Divine."*

## HANDS AND ARMS PAIN:
## "No matter how hard I try, I will never get what I desire."

**You continue to do good to others but you still feel unloved? Do you wonder why?**

You go beyond your capacity to fulfil the needs of your loved ones, but they take you for granted. They never value your efforts and hard work. They never return the same gesture back. You constantly feel that they do not love the way you love them. You try very hard to make your loved ones understand your feelings and emotions, but they fail to recognize your love. In fact, they feel that it is your duty to take care of them. Consequently, over a period of time, you feel a lack of love within and therefore, suffer with pains in your shoulders, hands and arms.

Another reason that can lead to pains in your hands and arms is when you set unreasonable goals for yourself in life. You work very hard to achieve your goals, but you are not able to achieve them. What happens when you try to swim against the waves of the ocean? Your shoulders, arms and hands feel very tired. You don't want to give up, so you constantly keep trying very hard to make your way against the flow but after some time, you feel very fatigued, miserable and lose hope. The pains in your hands and arms are only making you aware that you are trying very hard in your life. It is trying to warn you that you're going in the wrong direction. Wrong direction does not mean that you have taken a wrong route or your goals are wrong. It does not imply that your desires are not worth fulfilling. It simply means that you need to change. Change your thought process and your perspectives.

**Case Study**

Sameer came with the issue that he worked hard in his office, but his work was never appreciated. He was always blamed for being irresponsible. He felt that people didn't understand him. He had intense feelings of rejection. He also mentioned that he had conflicts with his younger brother. Although he loved him so much, but he always fought with him. He felt unwanted and unloved. He wanted to know, "What did I do, why am I always blamed, despite working so hard at work and in relationships?"

It was one the most rip-roaring therapy sessions that I came across in my practice. It resulted in a tremendous vortex of dormant emotions which triggered a dreadful past life. Gradually as the session continued, the dust settled, and the beads of the past got connected with the current life that brought immense clarity and self-realization. It was a long one and the most unforgettable session that will leave an indelible impact on your heart as well.

**Therapy Session:**

A deep hypnotic state was induced and therapy session began.

*Therapist: "What do you feel when you are blamed?"*

*Client: "I feel, what did I do?"*

*Therapist: "How does it make you feel?"*

*Client: "I feel very angry and helpless."*

*Therapist: "Repeat your statement: What did I do?"*

*Client: "What did I do? What did I do? What did I do?"*

*Client's hands started rising up in the air.*

*Therapist: "What is happening?"*

*Client cried: "I am feeling my both hands are rising up, I have no control."*

*Therapist: "What are you trying to do as your hands are rising up?"*

*Client: "I am asking for forgiveness from God."*

*Therapist: "Why are you asking forgiveness from God, what did you do?"*

*Client: "I don't know."*

*Therapist: "Where are you?"*

*Client: "I am in the water."*

*Client regressed to a past lifetime.*

*Therapist: "What are you doing there?"*

*Client: "I am dragging a woman in the water, she is drowning."*

*Therapist: "What are you feeling?"*

*Client: "I am very angry, I want to kill her."*

*Therapist: "Did she die?"*

*Client: "Yes... she is dead."*

*Therapist: "What happened later in that lifetime?"*

*Client: "I was blamed for killing her, I was rejected. I had to leave that place and go to the jungle to live."*

*It was noticed that he consciously stated these statements before the session began.*

*Therapist: "What are you feeling?"*

*Client: "I am feeling no one understands me."*

*Therapist: "What was the worst moment?"*

*Client: "I was feeling guilty, but still I was never accepted by the people and so I jumped into the well."*

*Client became restless. Pain in his lower back started and neck became stiff.*

*Therapist: "What are you feeling as you are dying?"*

*Client: "I am feeling very guilty and helpless."*

*Client felt vibrations in the feet and fingers.*

*Client's physical discomforts were healed and the past life closures were done, then the session continued.*

*Therapist: "In this current life when did that past life get triggered?"*

*Client: "I was 5 years old."*

*Therapist: "What happened when you were 5 years old?"*

*Client angrily exclaimed: "I drowned my 8 months old brother in the bathroom tub because my mother loved him more than me."*

*Therapist: "What happened next?"*

*Client: "My mother came and shouted at me."*

*Therapist: "What did you feel at that time?"*

*Client: "I felt unloved and rejected. My mother never understood my sentiments."*

*Therapist: "What did the child conclude?"*

*Client: "I have to love my brother to attract mothers love, so I decided to take care of him."*

*Pain in his shoulders and knees started.*

*Therapist: "Did you take care of him?"*

*Client: "Yes. Initially I was furious with him, but still cared for him helplessly."*

*Therapist: "Do you now understand why you are suffering from a pattern of being blamed?"*

*Client: "Yes."*

*Therapist: "Do you understand why you often have conflicts with your younger brother?"*

*Client: "Yes."*

*After deep introspection and self-realization, Client's shoulder and knee pains were healed and the 5 years old inner child was integrated with adult. Finally, the intense session came to an end.*

**Therapist Conclusion:**

After the session, Sameer consciously mentioned that he loved his brother, but as a child he had developed feelings of jealousy as mother took care of him more. As a child when he tried to kill the baby, his past life memory got triggered in which he had killed a woman in the same way. In that past life he had felt the same emotions of rejection and anger, and thus, the other beliefs of that past life also surfaced. As a result, unwavering emotions were amplified in his current life due to which he started feeling that people don't understand him and he was always blamed.

In his current life, Sameer had pain in his right arms because he felt unloved and rejected by his mother. His mother blamed him and made him feel guilty of trying to harm the baby. He felt his mother doesn't understand him and this belief kept on confirming later with other people in life, as he mentioned that people in his office blamed him and never understood him.

Further, Sameer decided to take the responsibility of the younger brother and take care of him, just because he thought that then his mother would love him and accept him. Responsibility was taken out of helplessness, rather than love. Pain always comes when there is guilt and feeling of helplessness. Therefore, he was suffering from pain in the shoulders and the lower back.

During the session he felt stiffness in the neck which clearly indicates that he was very stubborn and never understood anyone's perspective. He continued to feel angry and believed that other people including his brother, didn't understand him. He was never accepted. He was always blamed by them and although he took his responsibilities properly, he was never appreciated. Through the session he released a lot of suppressed emotions that were impacting his health and relationships. He gained profound insights and was able to evaluate the entire picture in an entirely new light of awareness and acknowledgment.

### Case Study: Hand Tremors and Shaking

Sunita, who was 30 years old felt tremors in her right hand when she was nervous or anxious, and gradually it was increasing. She wanted to heal the trembling hand as it caused embarrassment to her and she failed to find any conscious reason for her condition, so the transpersonal

Regression therapy session was conducted. It was an extremely overwhelming and heart touching session that led to an avalanche of immense emotions and unbelievable outcome.

**Therapy Session:**

Sunita was induced to a deep hypnotic state and the therapy session began.

*Therapist: "Is your hand shaking now?"*

*Client: "No."*

*Therapist: "Okay! So, close your eyes and go to the moment when for the first time you started feeling tremors in your hand."*

*The Client's hands started shaking.*

*Therapist: "What is happening?"*

*Client: "I feel pain in my right hand, as if someone is pulling my hand."*

*Therapist: "How old are you?"*

*Client cried: "I am 8 years old."*

*Therapist: "Why are you crying?"*

*Client: "My father is holding my right hand very tightly and hitting me with a hose pipe."*

*Therapist: "Why is he hitting you?"*

*Client: "I hit my brother, his tooth broke and he was bleeding?"*

*Client became restless and started moving her body. Her legs also started shaking.*

*Therapist: "What is happening?"*

*Client cried: "I am having a lot of pain in my hip and upper back."*

*Therapist: "What are you feeling?"*

*Client: "I am crying, I am yelling with pain, but he didn't stop."*

*Therapist: "What are you concluding as your father is hitting you?"*

*Client: "My parents love my brother only, they don't love me."*

*Therapist: "What was the worst moment?"*

*Client cried: "My mother kept seeing, but didn't save me."*

*Therapist: "How did this make you feel?"*

*Client: "I felt jealous of my brother. I hate him. But now I feel it was my mistake, I should not have hit him. I feel guilty. My mother also kept on saying that if I hurt him then I would be hit, so I tried not to commit any mistakes."*

*Therapist: "What changed in you after this?"*

*Client: "I started believing that if I commit any mistake, I will be hit. I started taking extra care in doing things as I was extremely terrified of being hit with a hose pipe."*

*Therapist: "How did this impact your life later?"*

*Client: "I started feeling anxious and nervous when I had to do things for other people. Like when guests came home, my hand used to shake. When I served them food, I felt tremors in my right hand. Whenever I felt that someone was watching me while I was cooking, I felt very nervous, so I preferred to cook alone. I felt a lot of tremors in my hand."*

*After deep introspection and self-realization, the 8 years old inner child was healed, and the old beliefs were changed. Then the physical discomforts were checked.*

*Therapist: "Are you still feeling any pains or tremors?"*

*Client: "No, I am fine, now."*

*Then the indelible session ended.*

**Therapist Conclusion:**

After the session, Sunita consciously told me that whenever she had to make important decisions in her life such as when buying a property, she felt tremors in her right hand, and she had difficulty in signing. It was concluded that it was the 8 years old Sunita, who was stuck in the traumatic memory of the past event and developed fears of committing mistakes. She consequently experienced hand tremors whenever she was afraid of being judged by others such as when guests were over, when she was cooking in presence of someone, or as her fear of being punished surfaced.

Your negative beliefs and emotions associated with traumatic past episodes continue to haunt you and impact your later life until you break the loop of the old patterns and heal yourself. Thus, it is essential to treat your physical symptoms by healing your subconscious mind, rather than suppressing your discomforts through medication.

## FINGER PAINS:

### "I need to grip control over every situation."

**Are you very organized? Do you want everything spick and span? Do you feel that you are one of those who appreciates perfection? Do you focus on very minute details while accomplishing your tasks?**

You tend to develop finger pains when you have a tendency of emphasizing too much on the minor details in everything that comes across you. You prefer flawlessness in everything that you possess or do in life. There is a need in you to keep your house and your work space very clean and in an organized manner.

Subconsciously, there is a need to control everything because you carry a very strong desire to be recognised by others. Thus, it makes you accomplish your tasks with perfection because there is a subconscious feeling of not good enough and lack of confidence in you. You keep on trying very hard to focus on the minute details, so that there is no scope of committing any mistakes or your work being rejected. The need for appreciation makes you do things perfectly and flawlessly. In some cases, it was observed that this need to be perfect led to immense fear of failure and fear of being judged.

For instance, there was a client who came to me with severe swelling and pains in her fingers of her right hand. After her session it was revealed that she had a fear of loud voices. Thus, she always made sure to complete all her tasks in time. She took care because she was scared of committing any mistakes. She was scared of loud voices and so she avoided being scolded by higher authorities. There was an inner child, 6 years old, who was stuck in the past memory, when her mother used to yell at her for her bad handwriting. It was the 6 years old child who developed, lack of confidence and feelings of not good enough because of her mother's expectations.

However, after the session, she consciously stated that she has very beautiful handwriting now. She added that because of her mother's aggressive behaviour, she turned into a perfectionist in her life. Her deeds were always recognized and people appreciated her later in her life. But negatively, she had developed fears of loud voices and need of recognition, which became a problem to her. She tried to control everything minutely and could not accept rejection. She developed false pride and she had two maintain that pride helplessly. She became workaholic. She tried to meet the deadlines and as a result she was under a lot of pressure and stress. There was a subconscious need in her to maintain false high standards that she had created for herself subconsciously.

After extensive research on all my clients who were suffering from finger pains and swellings, it displayed a very clear pattern of holding anger and grudges in their relationships. They were passive rebellions. Most of them were unaware of these emotions, and initially denied the concept. But after the therapy sessions they could connect the dots. They accepted the strong emotions that were suppressed in their subconscious memory. Precisely, every finger revealed their issues with different relationships in their life. Let's understand each finger in detail.

**Index Finger:** The pain in the index finger implies that you are facing issues with the dominating people in your life. It means that you are carrying subconscious fears and anger towards the authoritative figure in your life. This dominating person could be anyone currently present in your life, who would be triggering your horrified memories and suppressed emotions associated with some authoritative figure in your childhood.

**Middle Finger:** It is the tallest finger, so it implies issues with people with whom you have shared the longest time of your lifetime. You may be carrying very strong emotions associated with your parents or siblings.

**Ring Finger:** Pain in the ring finger means that you are facing problems with your spouse. You are subconsciously carrying some grudges or anger or guilt towards your spouse.

**Little Finger:** Little finger represents issues with the smallest relationship in your life. It could be your children or any new relatives, or friends. Pain in your little finger also implies that you consider yourself very fragile 'Touch me not' type of a person. It means that you are very sensitive at heart. To heal this pain, you just have to be strong and stand up for yourself.

**Thumb:** Thumb represents support. If you feel pain or get hurt in your thumb then it implies that you don't feel supported. It also conveys that you lack confidence and self-love.

Physical pains and emotional issues never develop overnight. The trigger is in the present, but the real root cause lies in your past.

**Healing of Hands, Arms and Fingers:**

**Self-realization:** Overview your life and focus on the benefits that each karmic teacher has helped you to achieve in your life. Think positive and practice gratitude and forgiveness. Try to see the bigger picture. Don't focus on the event or what harm did that person do to you. Think of all the strengths that you developed after that event.

**Change Your Perspective**: Stop controlling the situations. You don't need to take a lot of pressure and stress in order to control the outcomes. You can only work hard in your capacity. You don't have to impress anyone. Don't feel guilty over small mistakes, it is okay to commit mistakes. If you are not able to accomplish your desired results, avoid self-sabotaging yourself. It would only develop lack of confidence and low self-esteem in you. Never give up. Build your motivation, don't lose hope. Keep up the good work.

**Self-love:** Love and nurture yourself. Stop being so harsh on yourself. When you love yourself, then you emit a beautiful vibrating light of love towards others, which comes back to you in return in the same form of love. If you emit lack of love, then you will keep feeling that lack of love in your life because the lack will be returned to you. You must be aware of what goes around comes around. This law of attraction. Give and accept unconditional love.

**Chakras:** Throat chakra, heart chakra, and the solar plexus chakra get partially blocked or completely imbalanced because of your thought processes. You have to balance and activate these chakras in order to heal your pains in your hands and arms. You can read about this in detail under the Chakra section.

**Meditation:** To liberate oneself from entombed painful traumatic past memories and events, you can practice forgiving meditation in the book's "Healing" chapter. This will help you organically cure your subconscious mind and heal yourself from the inside out.

**Emotion Management Technique:** You can chant 'unloved' or 'sad' to surface the physical sensations, and then follow the EMT steps mentioned under the 'Emotion Management Techniques' section under the "Healing" Chapter of the book.

**Affirmations:**

*"I do in my capacity."*

*"I have set reasonable goals."*

*"I deserve the desired results."*

*"I feel confident to achieve my desired goals."*

*"I have faith in divine timing."*

*"I love and accept myself as I am."*

## HIP, THIGHS AND KNEE PAINS:
## "I have to defend myself, no one supports me."

Do you know that the Femur bone in your thighs that connects your hips to the knees, is the longest bone in your body? Majority of the cases who reported hip pains, thighs pains, sciatica and knee problems, had issues with their parents, siblings or other people with whom they shared the longest relationships in their life.

Do you feel unsupported? Do you feel that you only have to stand up and defend yourself just like an attorney as no one else will come and defend you? But have you noticed that in spite of you being so defensive, all your defences breakdown when your opponents are your own loved ones? You compromise helplessness for their sake, and that causes you pains or stiffness in your thighs, hips or knees.

**Case Study**

There was a client, Nirmal, who was 56 years old and complained of having pains in her thighs, often she suffered from aches in her hips. She had already tried several healing modalities like Ayurveda, Naturopathy and Physiotherapist, but they could only give her temporary relief and the pain continued to persist. So, she decided to seek transpersonal regression therapy to heal the root cause. As you read into the astonishing revelation, you will realise how your actions and words can affect your child's mental state.

**Therapy Session:**

The therapy session began after Nirmal was put into a profound hypnotic state.

*Therapist: "Are you feeling any pain right now?"*

*Client: "Yes, I am feeling pain in my right hip and I can feel some knots forming in both thighs, which are very painful."*

*Therapist: "How does that make you feel?"*

*Client: "I feel very helpless and frustrated. I feel why do I suffer from so many health problems? I wonder when is all this going to end?"*

*Therapist: "Just close your eyes and imagine these knots in your thighs. Give me your first impressions as to how they appear?"*

*Client: "They appear like small marbles/balls, scattered all over."*

*Clients pain in her hip intensified.*

*Therapist: "What is happening?"*

*Client: "I am feeling bad pain in my hip joint."*

*Therapist: "Go back in time to the first time ever, when you felt this bad pain so intensely that made you feel so helpless and frustrated. Give me your first impressions."*

*Client: "I am blank."*

*Therapist: "How old are you?"*

*Client: "I am 7 years old."*

*Therapist: "What happened when you were 7 years old?"*

*Client cried: "I was playing with small marble balls and my younger brother snatched them from me and scattered them all over. My mother was sleeping, so when she heard the noise, she woke up and came out. She scolded me and when I tried to explain that it was not my mistake, she slapped me."*

*Therapist: "How did that make you feel?"*

*Client: "I felt very angry over my mother. My mother was always biased. I felt so lonely and sad."*

*Therapist: "What did you conclude for yourself?"*

*Client: "I concluded that my parents always wanted a boy child. They preferred my brother over me. They never supported me."*

*Therapist: "How did you cope?"*

*Client: "I decided to stand up for myself."*

*Therapist: "How did this decision impact your later life?"*

*Client: "I decided to prove myself as the best child. I showed everybody that I was superior to my brother in every way. In fact, my parents now trust and value me more than my brother."*

*Therapist: "How is your relationship with your parents today?"*

*Client: "Oh, it's beautiful. I love them, I didn't even remember that event."*

*Therapist: "Now do you understand that it was the 7 years inner child who was stuck in the past and feeling the pain."*

*Client: "Yes."*

*Pains of Nirmal were healed during the session and the 7 years old inner child was integrated, and physical discomforts were checked.*

*Therapist: "Do you feel any discomfort?"*

*Client: "No."*

*The beautiful session then concluded with deep insights and wonderful self-realisation.*

**Therapist Conclusion:**

After the therapy session it was concluded that the 7 years old Nirmal was stuck in the past feeling that her parents were biased towards her as she was a girl, and they preferred a boy child. After the session, Nirmal consciously stated that her grandfather always said, "The legacy has to be carried out by the boy child." And thus, boys were always given preference in their family. She also added that as a child she felt that way, but as she grew up, she understood that her grandfather as well as her parents loved her more than her brother.

Consciously before the session when she was informed that hip pains and the thigh pains generally are suffered by people who have issues with their parents, she completely denied this fact arguing that she shared a wonderful relationship with her parents and siblings. But after the session, she was clear that it was the 7 years old inner child who was having issues with the parents and siblings. She mentioned that if she would not have taken the session then she would have never believed that she ever had any issues with her parents or siblings because they shared a very strong bond in the present.

Majority of my clients who suffered from hip and thigh pains, often developed sciatica pains.

## SCIATICA:
## "I cannot sit idle."

Sciatica pain is a shooting muscle pain from the hip through the thigh that goes down till the ankle. You develop sciatica pains when there is a need in you to keep yourself busy.

**Do you wonder why you cannot sit idle?**

If you are suffering from sciatica pains, then your mind is round the clock at work. Consequently, you feel physically as well as mentally tired. In some cases, it was observed that clients suffering from sciatica pains were not physically active, but they displayed a habit of continuous overthinking.

When you feel stuck in a never-ending loop of thought processes and mindset, then you try to keep yourself busy, to divert your mind. You want to just forget everything that keeps bothering you. And it is when you try to run from your plagued past memories, that you suffer from sciatica pain.

## KNEE PROBLEMS:
## "I can forgive but I can't forget."

**Do you feel that you have forgiven everyone who hurt you in the past?**

You have the impression that you have already moved on from the awful past memories, hurts, and scars, and that you have forgiven everyone who was responsible for your suffering. But the truth is that if you have knee problems, you are still caught in the past. Consciously, you feel that you have forgiven the people who caused you harm, but unconsciously, you suppress all the anger and resentment in your subconscious mind.

Your subconscious mind never forgets anything. Everything that you perceive through your five senses is stored as a memory in your subconscious mind. Your subconscious mind is your repository for all of your memories, good or bad. As a result, even if you forgive the people who hurt you, your subconscious mind remembers even minute details of every terrible experience. It recalls the exact words and acts of the people and stores them in the correct order. Your subconscious mind not only retains events and people, but it also stores your emotional reactions caused by those horrifying incidents, which continue to fire up in your present. As a result, despite your best efforts to ignore the traumatic experiences, your past continues to haunt you.

Through the case studies it was also observed the most of the clients who suffered with knee problems were very stubborn and displayed very rigid mindset. Following case study will help you to understand how your subconscious anger and stubbornness can be so painful physiologically.

**Case Study**

Kanak, 52 years old, was suffering from acute knee aches. She stated that something was present in her knees and that it moved when she walked. Doctors had advised her to proceed with the knee replacement surgery. Before undergoing the surgery, she opted to undergo the Regression Therapy to address the underlying reason for her knee problem. The shocking revelation through the session will cause you a wave of chills down your spine. It was a very heart touching session that I could never forget.

**Therapy Session:**

The therapy session began after Kanak was induced into a deep hypnotic trance state.

*Therapist: "Are you feeling knee pain right now?"*

*Client: "No, I'm on painkillers. I don't feel the pain right now."*

*Therapist: "Move your legs. Do you feel movement of anything present in your knees?"*

*Client: "Yes."*

*Therapist: "How does that make you feel?"*

*Client: "I feel very frustrated. I feel irritated. I want to know what is it that is stuck in my knee? I feel so helpless when it moves."*

*Therapist: "What are the doctors saying about this stuck thing present in your knees?"*

*Client: "I've got all the necessary medical diagnosis done, but doctors have no answer because they cannot see anything in my knees."*

*Therapist: "But you feel something is stuck?"*

*Client: "Yes."*

*Therapist: "How does this stuck thing make you feel?"*

*Client: "I feel confused and blank. I feel I have no control."*

*Therapist: "Go back in time to the moment when you felt so confused, helpless and blank; feeling loss of control."*

*Client started sobbing.*

*Therapist: "How old are you?"*

*Client: "I am 6 years old."*

*Therapist: "What happened when you were 6 years old?"*

*Client: "My father scolded me because I went out into the garden without taking his permission. He did not let me enter the house. He started yelling at me when I was climbing the stairs. I got scared and I urinated on the stairs."*

*Therapist: "How did that make you feel?"*

*Client: "I felt very confused and embarrassed as my neighbours came out of their house to check why my father was screaming. They saw my urine going down the stairs. My friends made fun of me."*

*Therapist: "How did that make you feel?"*

*Client: "I felt very angry over my father. I went into the room and locked myself."*

*Therapist: "When you locked yourself in the room, then what were you feeling?"*

*Client: "I felt very sad. I cried all night. Even my mother did not come to console me. I felt very lonely."*

*Therapist: "What did you conclude when your mother also did not come to console you?"*

*Client: "I concluded that no one loves me; I decided that when I grow big, then I will not listen to anyone."*

*Client cried out loudly: "Ah, ah..."*

*Therapist: "What happened?"*

*Client: "I'm feeling a lot of pain in my right knee."*

*Therapist: "What is it making you feel?"*

*Client: "I'm feeling very helpless, irritated and frustrated."*

*Therapist: "What changed in you after this incident?"*

*Client: "I stopped caring for my parents. I always used to do the opposite of whatever they asked me to do."*

*Therapist: "Do you feel that you turned into a passive aggressive child?"*

*Client: "Yes, I was very stubborn and loved isolation."*

*Therapist: "How is your relationship with your parents today?"*

*Client: "I am scared of my father as he is very dominating even today. But I know he loves and cares for me."*

*Therapist: "Do you understand how that incident impacted your little life as an adult?"*

*Client: "Yes, now I understand why I'm very stubborn."*

*Therapist: "Are you still feeling any pain or discomfort in your knees?"*

*Client: "No."*

*Therapist: "Do you still feel that there is something present in your knees? Please move your legs and check."*

*Client: "Right now when I move my legs, I don't feel anything in my knees, and nothing is moving.*

*The 6 years old child of Kanak was healed and integrated, and the session ended.*

**Therapist Conclusion:**

It was very clear from the session that the 6 years old inner child of Kanak was stuck in the past memory, feeling unloved, helpless and confused as her father scolded her outside the house. She got frightened and urinated on the staircase. She felt embarrassed as her neighbours and her friends saw her urine going down the stairs. Her father was very dominating. Hence, she became a passive aggressive child. She claimed that she did the exact opposite of whatever she was asked to do.

She accepted that she was very stubborn since then, and resisted change. After the session consciously Kanak told me that when she was very young, her parents used to leave her alone in the house every week as they went shopping. She told me that it was a Sunday evening when they were not in the house and she was feeling very bored, that is why she went to the garden to play without taking their permission. This incident emotionally affected the child and since then she became very defensive.

The child concluded that she was very young so she was weak at that age, but she decided that when she would grow old, she would take charge of her life. She also stated that her feelings of loneliness and unloved continued increasing in her later life. This happened because a loop was created in her mind due to the negative beliefs that she formed associated with that traumatic past episode. She added that she could not tolerate injustice and felt that she had to stand up for herself as no one would ever be there to support her.

People who have rigid mind sets suffer from neck pains, while those who feel unsupported often experience lower back pains. Kanak confirmed that she often suffered with neck ache and lower backache too.

**Healing Hip, Thigh, Sciatica and Knee Problems:**

Most importantly, accept change willingly and not helplessly.

**Forgiveness:** Forgive your past with understanding. Don't compromise for the sake of moving on. Think positive and analyse the benefits that you have gained from the past event and actions of the people involved. Remember that everything happens for a reason, and each individual in your life is only giving you certain lessons. Take all challenges as opportunities to learn, grow and become the most authentic part of you.

**Practice Gratitude:** Keep thanking everyone who has given you pain as well as love. Everyone who comes into your life is your well-wisher and not your enemy.

**Chakras:** Root chakra and sacral chakra are imbalanced. When you feel that you are not supported in life then your root chakra gets partially or completely blocked. It results in anxiety, fear and insecurities. You feel sad and frustrated due to which your sacral chakra also gets imbalanced. To heal your hip, thigh, sciatica and knee problems, you need to feel grounded and trust everyone around you. Trust people around you and stop proving yourself. Turn inwards to feel peace. You can refer to the chakra section of the book under the "Healing" Chapter to heal and balance your Chakras. You can also do Chakra meditations and activate your chakras through mantras.

**Meditation:** To liberate oneself from entombed painful traumatic past memories and events, you can practice meditation in the book's "Healing" Chapter. This will help you heal your subconscious mind deeply.

**Emotion Management Technique:** You can chant 'unsupported' or 'helpless' to surface the physical sensations and then follow the EMT steps mentioned under the "Emotion Management Techniques" section under the "Healing" Chapter of the book.

## LEG PROBLEMS:
## "I am always stuck in 'What if? mindset."

**Do you have fear of moving ahead in life? Are you overthinking about some new projects or new career? When you have to make**

**important decisions, then you feel pains, heaviness or stiffness in your legs, calf, ankle, feet (sole, bridge area) or toes.**

Repeated leg problems are caused when there is tremendous fear of future. When your finances are at stake or when you are stuck in stressful relationships then you feel anxious in making important decisions. This anxiety causes heaviness or pain in your legs. Even in case of injuries, if you get hurt in your legs then it implies that you are carrying subconscious fears of moving ahead in life. When you have experienced past failures then you develop subconscious anxiety which continue to resurface in your present. Thus, it is not a coincidence if you get hurt in your ankle, toes or knees. However, different parts of your legs indicate specific emotional causes of struggles in life.

**Calf**: Calf problems indicate that your failures in the past are causing you extreme anxiety and nervousness. If you experience calf pains or stiffness, it could suggest that you have made decisions in the past that did not turn out to be potent. As a result, subconscious fear or guilt may reemerge when you have to make new decisions for the future. Consequently, you feel discomfort in your calves.

**Ankle**: Not feeling supported in your decisions that leads to tremendous fear of moving ahead in life. You feel helpless and anxious of making important decisions as no one supports you. Financial instabilities and insecurities.

**Feet**

**Sole**: Not feeling grounded; physical and emotional instability. Living in fantasies or an illusionary world. Trying to run away from reality. You feel helpless and stuck in your financial conditions as well as relationships.

**Bridge**: Letting others step on your feet. This means that you are letting other people interfere in your life. You feel insecure and helpless of taking drastic life changing decisions thus you continue to tolerate other people's disrespectful behaviour and remain stuck in the relationship silently.

**Toes**: Excessive focusing on the minute details. Maybe you are working very hard in your life, but you are focusing too much on minute details due to which your toes start aching or you may feel sensations in your toes. When you are going through financial or relationship insecurities then you continue to suppress your anger, anxiety and helplessness in your toes, as a result you experience pain or may hurt them unconsciously.

**Case Study**

Soham, 35 years old, lamented the fact that he was always dependent on his relatives for his living. He intended to start a business on his own, but he was never successful. He complained of acute leg heaviness and a continuous ache in his right ankle. He felt bewildered and pondered why couldn't he do his business independently. Over time, he had developed the beliefs of not being good enough and a lack of confidence, which drove him to seek counselling. Therefore, Transpersonal Regression Therapy was conducted, in which he regressed into his past lifetime which connected all the dots of his current life beautifully as it unfolded. It was a very intriguing and satisfying session and will flabbergast you.

**Therapy Session:**

Soham was induced into a deep hypnotic trance state and the therapy session began.

*Therapist: "Do you feel any pain in your legs right now?"*

*Client: "No."*

*Therapist: "How does it make you feel when you are dependent on relatives for your living?"*

*Client: "I feel useless, frustrated and irritated. Sometimes I feel very angry with myself?"*

*Client began to experience bodily discomfort.*

*Therapist: "What is happening?"*

*Client: "I'm feeling my both legs have become very heavy and numb."*

*Therapist: "Are you able to move your legs?"*

*Client: "No, they have become absolutely numb. I cannot move them."*

*Therapist: "How does this make you feel?"*

*Client: "I'm feeling stuck."*

*Therapist: "How does it make you feel, when you're stuck?"*

*Client: "I feel helpless."*

*Therapist: "Go back to the first time you felt helpless because you couldn't move as your legs had become absolutely numb. Get all the impressions and let me know."*

*Client: "I can see myself on the road. I feel this is me, but I have never seen this road."*

*Client regressed to his past life.*

*Therapist: "Get clear impressions of what you are doing on the road?"*

*Client: "I can see blood all around me, and my legs and lower body are terribly damaged."*

*Therapist: "Go to a few moments before the injury occurs."*

*Client: "I see myself strolling down the street with two large bags. I'm wearing headphones connected to a Walkman. I'm feeling cheerful, but then a car smashes me from behind."*

*Therapist: "As the car smashes you, look around and describe exactly what you are feeling and what happens next?"*

*Client: "I can see blood all around me and I am not able to get up. I am not able to move. My body has become very heavy. I'm feeling very restless, very anxious and helpless as there is no one to help me. I'm crying for help, but there is no one. I feel I will die."*

*Therapist: "Did you die there?"*

*Client: "Yes, I can see my dead body."*

*Therapist: "Just a few moments before you were dying, get all the impressions of your dying thoughts."*

*Client: "I was thinking that I will not be able to move now ever in my life. I will always be dependent on others as my legs are crushed badly. I was feeling terrified with the thought that I will become a handicap."*

*Therapist: "That life is now over and it bears absolutely no influence in your current life."*

*Therapist: "When did that past life trigger in your current life? Let me know, how old were you?"*

*Client: "I was 17 years old."*

*Therapist: "What happened when you were 17 years old?"*

*Client: "I recall hurting my right ankle badly while playing football. My ligament was ripped, and I was bedridden for 6 months."*

*Therapist: "Get all of your impressions and thoughts from the period you were bedridden."*

*Client: "Oh, I felt so miserable. I could not walk, I felt like a handicap. I couldn't even walk to the toilet by myself. I was so dependent. I was so angry with myself at times when I felt helpless and stuck on the bed. I couldn't move on my own, and I was irritable and frustrated as I had to wait for someone to carry me to the toilet. This memory terrifies me. I don't even want to recall it. I was in an awful situation."*

*These thoughts were similar to what he felt in the past lifetime before dying.*

*Therapist: "How long were you dependent on others?"*

*Client: "For about 3 months."*

*Therapist: "Were you okay after that, and able to walk on your own?"*

*Client: "Yes, I could finally walk on my own, and I felt so glad that I could finally enjoy my life."*

*Therapist: "Get all your impressions and thoughts when you were dependent on others."*

*Client: "I used to feel terrible depending on others for petty things. I wondered how long I would be stuck in that bed."*

*Therapist: "Now do you understand how your past life got triggered due to your leg injury?"*

*Client: "Yes."*

*The adult gained wisdom through self-realization, and the 17 years old inner child of Soham was healed and integrated.*

*Therapist: "Now do you understand how your 17 years old inner child's conclusions and thoughts made you dependent on others."*

*Client: "Yes, now I understand."*

*Therapist: "Just check, do you still feel numbness or heaviness in your legs, now?"*

*Client: "No."*

*Therapist: "Do you feel any other discomfort in your physical body?"*

*Client: "No, I'm absolutely fine."*

*It was a very lengthy session, but Soham found all the answers to his questions that made his heart ponder. After deep introspection and healing, the amazing session ended.*

**Therapist Conclusion:** It was concluded through the session that when Soham was 17 years old as a result of the leg injury, his past life got triggered in which he died in a car accident. In his current life, his dying thoughts were the trigger for his mental condition while he was suffering from intense pain and similar mental stress of being bedridden and feeling helpless of being dependent on others. As a result, he was imprisoned in his past. Despite the fact that he had recovered from the physical injuries, the mental trauma of that past life was triggered. Thus, all of his negative beliefs about being dependent on others and emotions linked to that episode resurfaced. Consequently, subconsciously he felt dependent on people for his living. This amplified the similar emotions throughout those 6 months of pain and dependency and he continued to suffer later in his life. Although he had physically recovered, his mind remained stuck in his past.

Therefore, it is essential to keep your mind free from negative thoughts. It's easier said than done but it's true. You never know which negative thought or beliefs may trigger your horrified past and increase your sufferings. Let's learn how to avoid heal leg issues.

**Healing Leg and Feet Problems:**

**Transpersonal Regression Therapies:** Therapies are the fastest way to cure your leg problems as they can help you to identify your subconscious real reasons for pain or heaviness. Once you heal your past, you will notice tremendous improvement not only in your leg problems as well as financial conditions.

**Avoid Overthinking:** To heal your leg and feet problems, you have to avoid overthinking. Before taking major decisions, carefully analyse all the pros and cons and move ahead confidently. Don't let your past failures hold you back. Seek approval from others but take decisions based on your conscience. Follow your instincts and make wise decisions.

**Be Realistic:** Avoid fantasizing and stay in reality. Be like a man of actions, not only words. It is good to make strategies, but it is equally important to implement your ideas. Do not feel scared of bringing your thoughts into actions. Believe in yourself.

**Chakras:** Balance your root chakra and sacral chakra. When you feel extreme fear and anxiety or helplessness due to financial insecurities, then your root chakra gets either partially blocked or completely blocked. As a result, you often feel dissatisfied and frustrated. Consequently, your sacral chakra also gets blocked which leads to relationship conflicts too. Your professional life as well as personal life gets messy. Hence, it is very essential for you to activate your root chakra and the sacral chakra. You can refer to the Chakra section of the book under the "Healing" Chapter to heal and balance your chakras. You can also do chakra meditations and activate your chakras through mantras.

**Meditation:** To liberate oneself from entombed painful traumatic past memories and events, you can practice meditations in the book's "Healing" Chapter. This will help you heal your subconscious mind deeply.

**Emotion Management Technique:** You can chant 'restless', 'anxiety', 'unsupported' or 'helpless' to surface the physical sensations and then follow the EMT steps mentioned under the "Emotion Management Techniques" section in the "Healing" Chapter of the book.

## BACK PROBLEMS:
## "I need support and movement in my life."

You feel stuck in your daily routine. You lack excitement and creativity that leads to boredom. Your subconscious mind triggers you to bring change in way of your living, but you feel anxious and unsupported in your decisions. The previous financial set backs or life situations hold you back from moving ahead confidently, as a result, you feel helpless and stuck in your situation. However, each part of your back hurts due to some particular emotional reasons, as you will read further, you will understand this in detail.

### Upper Backaches: Are you taking over burdens of responsibility?

Upper back is that portion where we pick up weights. Hence, it is very simple to understand the root cause for your upper back swelling, stiffness or aches. It signals that you are weighing yourself down with a lot of burdens of responsibilities. Taking care of your loved ones is good, but overdoing or taking loads of responsibilities will lead to upper back pains. If you are taking the burdens of your loved ones just because it is your duty, then you will often feel helpless. When you will do anything with helplessness, then you will suffer with aches and pains.

### Middle Back Aches: Do you feel guilty for not being able to fulfil your responsibilities properly?

Majority of the people who suffer with the middle back pains often experience pains or stiffness in their upper back as well. You feel a shooting pain starting from your upper back which continues to your middle back. This pain arises when you are unable to bear the burdens of your responsibilities. You are afraid of losing your relationship or a loved one and as a result, you continue to execute your tasks helplessly. Finally, you feel guilty when you are weary and unable to accomplish your tasks. Fear and guilt are the major emotions which are the root cause of middle backache.

**Lower Backaches: Do you feel unsupported by your loved ones?**

If you're suffering from the lower back aches, then, you may be feeling unsupported by the people around you. Backbone is our rock foundation. It is the unit of support that holds our entire body together. Hence, when you feel that your ideas and actions are not accepted by the people you value, then you feel frustrated, disappointed and unhappy. Consequently, your vibrations become very low as a result, you feel very helpless and insecure in your life. This affects your relationships at deeper levels which causes you extreme fear and anxiety. Thus, you suffer from extreme lower back pains.

This situation is even worse for you if you are a provider. Mental and emotional distress not only impacts your health but barges your professional life as well and soon, you find yourself in financial debts. It is observed that when you experience financial instabilities or when your finances are stuck, then also you tend to develop back pains or you may attract scenarios, in which you hurt your back.

**Tailbone pain: Do you feel that you are stuck in life?**

You may be stuck physically, emotionally, or mentally, if you are suffering from tailbone pains. Majority of my clients who were suffering from the tailbone pains were stuck in their old painful memories. As a result, not only were they suffering from lower back pains, they also had stomach issues. Most of them stated that they had invested huge amounts, although they were not consciously worried about their finances but through their therapy sessions, it was discovered that the root cause of their lower back pain was financial stress as their mind was constantly stuck in "What if?"

You cannot fool your mind, most of the clients claimed that they were leading a very happy and prosperous life but if you are suffering from severe back pains then that implies the root cause of your suffering lies in the past. There may be certain rigid beliefs formed in the past that are causing you pain in your present. Lower back pains are often experienced when you are struggling in your finances and relationships.

In both scenarios you need movement; a change in perspective. When you start flowing with an open mindset, then you will notice the flow in your money and relationships, but when you are stuck in your stern belief patterns then you will suffer from stiffness in your lower back and also feel stuck in both finances and relationships.

**Case Study: Severe Lower Back pain**

Nita, who was 42 years old, complained of severe back pain. She told me that since she had booked the therapy session, she was feeling pain in her right hand elbow too. She wanted to know why was she suffering with severe body pains and diseases always. It was a tedious session that paced back and forth between the past and present lives, but it eventually resulted in a satisfactory resolution and release from the traumatic past. This session will assist you in understanding how physical injuries from our previous lives may be carried forward into our present lives in the form of cellular memories that influence your current life if triggered by your negative thought processes.

**Therapy Session:**

Nita was induced a deep trance state and the therapy commenced.

*Therapist: "Feel your pains, back pain and arm pain, which one is the worst?"*

*Client: "I am having back pain but in my right arm elbow, it's unbearable right now."*

*Therapist: "How is it making you feel?"*

*Client: "I feel as if it's badly wounded, maybe it's cut."*

*Therapist: "Breathe into this part of your body and feel this pain growing."*

*Client: "It's paining very badly, my head is spinning. I am feeling dizzy."*

*Clients body language changed. Client started feeling breathless and hands started shaking.*

*Therapist: "What is happening?"*

*Client: "I am falling down."*

*Therapist: "Where have you landed?"*

*Client: "I am on the ground."*

*Client became very uncomfortable and started shaking.*

*Therapist: "Any physical sensation?"*

*Client: "I am having a lot of pain in my right hand, headache and extreme back pain."*

*Therapist: "Describe the ground where you landed."*

*Client: "The ground is rough and made up of rocks. My lower back collided with the earth and landed on the rocks. I am feeling unbearable pain in my full body, especially my lower back."*

*Therapist: "Where did you fall from?"*

*Client: "From the mountain cliff. It was extremely high and deep."*

*Client started choking suddenly.*

*Therapist: "What is happening, how did you fall down?"*

*Client cried: "Someone is trying to suffocate me, he has caught hold of my neck very tightly and pushed me."*

*Therapist, "Did you roll down or fall down straight on the ground?"*

*Client: "It is a green mountain. I got stuck in the cone shaped trees and then fell on the ground."*

*Client's hands started shaking continuously and she started crying loudly.*

*Client: "I can't see my right hand on the body!"*

*Therapist: "See the whole scene in slow motion and figure out what happened?"*

*Client: "My right hand was cut by the sharp edge of the tree because my body struck it first, when I was thrown off the cliff. I am feeling a severe headache, I will die now."*

*Therapist: "Did you die?"*

*Client: "Yes, but after a long time."*

*Client cried, "I am feeling a lot of pain in my neck and lower back."*

*Therapist: "What are you feeling before dying?"*

*Client: "I am feeling stuck in pain and helpless."*

*Therapist: "What are your last thoughts?"*

*Client: "Why did this person do this to me? I will never forgive him."*

*The client was healed and the file of the traumatic past life was closed.*

*Therapist: "In this present life, when did that past life get triggered?"*

*Client: "When I was 27 years old."*

*Therapist: "What happened when you were 27 years old?"*

*Client: "I picked up my 8 months old child and I suddenly got a back pain, and my body got a paralytic attack. I was bedridden."*

*Therapist: "What did you feel at that time?"*

*Client: "I felt stuck in pain, and I felt helpless for a long time."*

*Same emotions were triggered, which she felt in that past life when she had hit on the rough ground.*

*Therapist: "How long were you in pain?"*

*Client: "I suffered from a slipped disc, it took 2 months, then I was fine."*

*After the deep introspection by the adult Nita and self-realization, the inner child was healed and the lengthy session finally came to an end.*

**Therapist Conclusion:**

After the session, Nita consciously mentioned that when she was 27 years old, she had shifted to a new place as her husband was posted there. She was unhappy, moreover, she delivered the second baby at that time, and she felt unsupported in the new place. She had to take care of everything on her own and the responsibilities of the two children single handedly in the new environment.

As I had mentioned earlier, the root cause for lower back ache is feeling unsupported and helpless. Nita was feeling exactly the same emotions during that time and thus, she suffered from the issue of slip disc.

Further, in the past life, Nita died with intense body pains, especially in her lower back as she hit on the rocks with intense pressure and her right hand got cut by the tree. Therefore, in her current life when that past life got triggered, she suffered with acute back pain and paralytic attack in her lower body till legs. Since her mind was stuck in the question, "Why did he do this to me, I will never forgive him!" Nita, in her current life, suffered from a migraine attack soon after that past life got triggered at the age of 27. As you are now aware, migraine occurs when your half consciousness is stuck somewhere in the past. As Nita's right arm was cut in the past, when her memory of that terrible past life triggered, she started suffering from migraine attacks also.

Nita testified after a few weeks that her right arm pain and back pains were cured and she also added in her review that she used to have pain in her feet, which also was completely gone after the session. She also stated that she wanted to start her own business but was unable to do so due to her physical ailments. She began her own trading business after the therapy session and was living an abundant life.

Regression Therapy sessions heal you deeply and bring remarkable results in health and relationships. The astounding outcomes of the session can be witnessed immediately after the profound awareness and deep healing, which leads to everlasting changes in your life.

**Healing Backaches**

**Healing Upper Back Aches and Middle Back Aches:**

To heal your upper back aches and middle back aches, you have to balance your heart chakra and solar plexus chakra. Avoid self-criticism and guilt. Remember that you can do only in your capacity for others. Avoid self-sabotaging yourself by taking over burdens of responsibilities. You are scared of loss of control, and as a result you don't trust people around you. Accept and give love unconditionally. People around you are not as bad as you think. If you had issues in some relationships in the past, that does not mean that you cannot be happy in other new relationships.

Everyone comes into your life for a reason, so the learning is different from each one. People with whom you have problems are generally, your karmic teachers, they teach you your life lessons with bitterness. However, there are soul group connections and soulmates, who come into your life to teach you with love. Until you dive into the relationship, you will never be able to find out who is your karmic teacher, and who is your soul connection. So just be open to give and receive unconditional love.

If you are suffering from the upper back aches, then you may be having weak throat chakra as well. When you have communication issues within your relationships then your throat chakra gets blocked. Try to communicate clearly. Don't suppress your thoughts and emotions. It is okay to express. Try it!

**Healing Lower Back Ache and Tail Bone Pains:**

Transpersonal Regression Therapies is the fastest way to heal you pains as it helps you to become aware of the negative stern beliefs subconsciously stored during your past. However, at your level also you can heal your pains, if you can identify the primary reason of your stuck mindset. Just acknowledgement and acceptance can heal you. You have to avoid being rigid. When you will become flexible, you will observe the positive flow in every aspect of your life, not only health but also in your finances and relationships.

When you are suffering from lower back ache and tail bone pains, then your solar plexus chakra, as well as your sacral chakra and the root chakra are either partially blocked or completely blocked. You have to take charge of your life. Feel your power and creativity. Avoid dwelling into the past and feeling guilt. Liberate yourself from the unwanted thoughts and emotions which are no longer serving you. Remember, you are the source of your own happiness, so don't depend on anyone to make you feel happy.

Life is not good or bad, it is how you feel it. Happiness will only come to you only when you are willing to be happy, so take charge of your happiness. Let go of your past. Forgive yourself and forgive the people around you. You suffer from tailbone pains when you are stuck in your rotten past memories.

Complete your life purpose. Don't feel anxious about implementing new ideas. Believe in yourself and move ahead confidently. Don't let your past failures hold you back. Life gives you ups and downs, but there is duality on Earth. Change is inevitable. So, nothing will be permanent. Don't get disheartened by the dark nights. It is said, "It is darkest before the dawn." Don't give up.

Keep moving to succeed in life. Success in literal sense may not mean being successful in whatever you do. When you don't give up and keep moving, you will definitely succeed in completing all your life lessons, which your soul has chosen before taking birth on Earth. Ultimately, that is your sole mission and life purpose.

To heal your back problems, you can recite affirmations as well as there are other ways of activating your throat chakra, heart chakra, solar plexus chakra, sacral chakra, and root chakra, which you can refer to under the Chakra section in the "Healing" Chapter of the book.

Meditation: To bring peace of mind and relieve stress you can practice meditations in the book's "Healing" Chapter. This will help you heal your subconscious mind deeply.

Emotion Management Technique: You can chant 'restless', 'anxiety', 'unsupported' or 'helpless' to surface the physical sensations and then follow the EMT steps mentioned under the "Emotion Management Techniques" section under the "Healing" Chapter of the book.

# *Chapter 13*
# GENITALS

## VAGINA AND UTERUS ISSUES:
## "My partner doesn't support me in front of his parents."

**Do you feel annoyed over your husband? Or do you feel that he supports and loves his mother or both parents more than you?**

If you are suffering from burning sensations or rashes in your vagina, white discharge issues or uterus related problems like endometriosis, irregular menstrual cycles, excessive bleeding or menopausal issues, then you are most probably carrying rage towards your spouse. Maybe today the relationship between you and your spouse would be fine, but these vaginal or uterus issues are caused due to the unhealed suppressed emotions of traumatic episodes in your past.

For example, 48 years old Mehek was suffering from endometriosis and heavy bleeding issues. A Transpersonal Regression Therapy session was done to heal the root cause. During the session, Mehek regressed to her age of 23, to the moment when she chose to marry Prakash against the will of her parents. But after her marriage, it came to her surprise that her beloved Prakash did not support her. Whenever she faced any issues with her in-laws, especially her mother-in-law, her husband always supported his mother, even if she was wrong. While they were in the room, he always asked Mehek to understand the situation and amend her mistakes. Mehek used to feel furious by the behaviour of her husband. For a few years, she felt very helpless and did not complain, but finally, she decided to stand up for herself.

48 years old Mehek mentioned that currently, her relationship with her in-laws and husband was fine but it was the 23 years old Mehek who was stuck feeling rage over the husband. It was clear that Mehek was suffering from endometriosis because she felt that her husband did not support her when she needed him the most. As mentioned in the back pain section, when you feel unsupported, then you suffer from lower back pains as well as abdominal issues. Consciously after the session, Mehek reported that she was suffering from intense tailbone pains and gas issues also. After the successful session, Mehek emailed a letter of gratitude in which she mentioned that her bleeding stopped after just one session and her gas pains and tail bone pains also vanished.

Menopausal symptoms like excessive or continuous, unstoppable bleeding occurs when you hide anguish and rage towards your husband. However, endometriosis and other uterus related issues like cysts or fibroids were also reported by the majority of my clients who displayed a pattern of resentment towards their mother, siblings as well as kids also.

Another interesting fact that was discovered through the research was that if you develop painful bruises or dryness around your vaginal area, then that implies that you are carrying guilt towards your husband. Do you keep secrets from your husband? What are you hiding from your husband? Think about it.

For instance, a client experienced white discharge, which caused inflammation between her vaginal area and thighs (panty line). She had tried numerous medications, ointments and healing modalities but her suffering continued, therefore she wanted to heal the root cause through the Regression Therapy. She saw herself heading down the stairs during her trance session. Her feet twisted unexpectedly and she slipped. She was not wounded, though, since she grabbed the railing. I inquired, "What does it remind you of?" She replied in a glum tone, "After my marriage, I fell in love with a young man. Oh! I feel terrible. I mean, how could I have done this to my husband? This thought is awful. I was drawn to his charming appearance and could not control my feelings.

Jesus, he was so adorable. I knew it was morally and ethically wrong to fall for a stranger, when I was already committed to someone else. Although I did not cheat on my husband, it was just a fling. But I still feel guilty for thinking about someone else and hiding it from him. I feel ashamed for deceiving him. My husband is a gem of a person and I love him madly. I don't know how I got attracted to that young chap? God forgive me for my sin."

After a long pause I asked, "Just try to recall, did you develop this white discharge issue or vaginal problems after that incident?" She replied, "Yeah, but not immediately; maybe after a year or so."

Therapist Conclusion: Client was unambiguously in pain as a result of her shame and guilt. Vagina is your private part. It is a part which you hide from people. It is associated with shame. The client was experiencing feelings of remorse and regret because of her shameful act of keeping secret from her husband, as a result, she developed issues in her vagina.

**Healing of Vaginal and Uterus Problems:**

Solar plexus chakra as well as sacral chakra and the root chakra are either partially blocked or completely blocked. you must learn to forgive your family members. Forgiving has the potential to help you in releasing yourself from the shackles of your horrendous past.

Uterus is the symbol of divine feminine energy. Each individual carries both divine feminine and divine masculine energy. Feminine energy is the energy to love and nurture yourself, while the divine masculine energy is to serve others. Your family means the world to you. You have devoted your entire self to your loved ones, and in doing so, you have forgotten yourself completely. As a result, your divine masculine energy has increased which created an imbalance in your own energy system.

You need to balance your divine feminine energy and masculine energy. Practice self-love. Self-love is not selfishness. You can love yourself as well as take care of the other people around you with the same love and compassion. Don't be hard on yourself. Don't punish yourself. You don't have to be a perfectionist. Nobody is perfect and nobody needs to be. Instead, overview your life. Review all your hardships as an opportunity to do things better in the future without blaming yourself and others for how your life has been so far. Applaud for yourself for coming so far. Appreciate yourself and recognize your own efforts. Embrace your inner strength. Don't let your frustrations suppress your creativity. Let your creative ideas fly high and make you shine. Unravel the tapestry of your true identity and potential. Unearth the hidden facets of yourself. Remember, you are the creator of your own destiny. Love and accept yourself as you are. Feel worthy and deserving.

*"Happiness is just like a butterfly, when you chase, it is always beyond your grasp, but if you sit quietly, it may alight upon you."*

You can refer to the chakra section of the book under the "Healing" Chapter to heal and balance your chakras. You can also do chakra meditations and activate your chakras through mantras.

Meditation: To liberate oneself from entombed painful traumatic past memories and events, you can practice meditations in the book's "Healing" Chapter. This will help you heal your subconscious mind deeply. These meditations will help you in forgiveness and healing your physical issues.

Emotion Management Technique: You can chant 'anger', 'anxiety', 'unsupported' or 'helpless' to surface the physical sensations and then follow the EMT steps mentioned under the "Emotion Management Techniques" section under the "Healing" Chapter of the book.

## PENIS ISSUES:
## "I feel disappointed and dissatisfied by my life."

Clients who suffered with penile issues displayed a common pattern of being dissatisfied. They were mostly introvert during their childhood. They had lack self-confidence and found difficult to express their emotions, as a result, they suffered from penile problems like erectile dysfunction, ejaculation problems, balanitis and other penile conditions or diseases, and even low sperm count.

There was unconsciously suppressed performance anxiety and tremendous fear of failure in cases of low sperm count or erectile dysfunctions. They felt nervous when they met new people and also carried intense fear of being judged. Due to some past humiliating or embarrassing events that occurred in their life, they developed subconscious feelings of shame and guilt, which triggered during sexual performance, consequently causing them anxiety that affected their sexual life.

In majority of clients, it was observed that during their childhood their mind was set with a belief that they were a source to maintain the legacy of their family. All of them displayed immense subconscious fear and pressure of upholding the dignity and pride of their family by giving birth to a boy child and being extremely successful in life. As a result, they suffered with penile issues. In most cases the issue was only these distorted beliefs and suppressed fear that was blocking their success and in a few cases, obstructing their desire to become a father.

Penile issues were frequently found in people who were going through an arduous period in their lives. They were mostly stressed because of financial insecurities or a quarrel in their relationships. They experienced very challenging situations in their relationships as well as finances. The uphill battle that they were fighting often led to intense psychological pressures and anxiety which in turn interrupted their brain from sending signals to their penis. This resulted in inadequate blood flow, resulting in unsatisfactory sexual performance. Consequently, they suffered from sexual frustrations and dissatisfaction. They also developed inferiority complex as well as feelings of not good enough, which resulted in low self-esteem.

**Case Study**

Priyank, who was 38 years old complained of having erectile dysfunction and wanted to seek the therapy session. Before the therapy session he mentioned that he had a huge financial loss a year ago and was suffering from depression. He had been seeking psychological counselling and was on anxiety pills. During the therapy session, Priyank regressed to his age of 14, when he was in 9th grade.

**Therapy Session:**

*While talking Priyank started sweating, hence the therapy session started immediately without any trance state.*

*Therapist: "Why are you sweating?"*

*Client: "I am locked in the basement."*

*Therapist: "Who has locked you in the basement?"*

*Client: "My father."*

*Therapist: "Why?"*

*Client: "Because I didn't score well in my exams."*

*Therapist: "What are you feeling?"*

*Client: "I am very scared; I wonder how long I will be punished. It's very dark and hot in the basement and there are rats. It's badly stinking and it feels so filthy."*

*Therapist: "What did you do then?"*

*Client: "I kept crying, yelling, but no one heard me. I felt so helpless, so weak, but I could not do anything."*

*Therapist: "How long were you stuck in the basement?"*

*Client: "For about two hours."*

*Therapist: "In those two hours, just get an impression of your thoughts and emotions."*

*Client: "I was feeling very angry over my father, and I decided that I will never score well in my exams if he continues to punish me in this manner."*

*Therapist: "Did you score less in your next exams?"*

*Client: "Yes. I failed in my next exams to destroy his false pride."*

*Therapist: "Did your father lock you in the basement at that time also?"*

*Client: "No, he sent me to the hostel."*

*Therapist: "What did you feel when he sent you to the hostel?"*

*Client: "Oh, I felt extremely sad and lonely, but I had no other option. I completely gave up. I knew that there was no point in explaining my feelings to my father. For him scoring good marks were more important than his son. He could go to any extent to maintain his false pride."*

*Therapist: "How is your relationship with your father today?"*

*Client: "Today, it's absolutely fine. I am surprised how this episode is the root cause of my sexual problem."*

*Therapist: "Do you now understand how the stubbornness of the 14 years old inner child's choice to fail in his performances, affected your sexual life in adolescence."*

*Client sighs: "Yes."*

*After the deep introspection and self-realization, the 14 years old inner child of Priyank was healed and the beautiful session ended.*

**Therapist Conclusion:**

It was very clear that when Priyank was 38 years old, he had subconsciously suppressed rage for father that turned him into a rebellion. He developed passive aggressive behaviour and decided to sabotage himself as well as his father to destroy his father's false pride by failing in his exams. Consequently, his decision to perform adversely continued and led to lack of confidence, low self-esteem, feelings of inadequacy and incompetence. During intercourse, the semen triggered his repressed memory of being locked in the basement making him feel dirty, stinky and filthy in the same way, and therefore, he could not enjoy his sex life. Although his relationship with his father was fine in the present, it was the 14 years old inner child of Priyank who remained stuck in the past memory. After the shocking revelation through the intense and lengthy session, the adult Priyank gained self-realization and was liberated from his traumatic past. After a few days, he emailed a note expressing his gratitude for curing his penile condition in just one session.

## PROSTATE DISEASES:
## "I feel rejected by my loved ones."

Prostate is a part of the male reproductive organ which includes the penis, seminal vesicles and testicles. It is a gland that surrounds the urethra. It is like a tube, the size of a walnut, through which urine passes out of the body. Prostate symptoms could be pain, burning sensations or blood while passing urine. Urinary Tract Infection (UTI) occurs in men due to longer length of urethra and because of the prostatic fluid. The prostatic fluid carries antibacterial properties due to which it prevents bacteria from growing, as a result, it increases the chances of urinary infection in men. Common symptoms are intense pain, urgent and frequent urination. It was observed that the primary cause of prostate diseases and UTI in men was extreme anger, especially over their wife and children.

People who suffered from prostate disease felt rejected by their loved ones. They were well disciplined men, who followed rules and regulations and expected others around them to also follow them and thus they were perceived as a dominating personality. Root cause of the prostate problems is suppressed anger and resentment. Repeated misunderstandings and conflicts with not only their loved ones but with other people in the surroundings also was the cause of their Prostate disease. Prostate never develops overnight, it is a long term deeply repressed anger, so it's essential to keep the anguish in control. *Precaution is better than cure.*

**Case Study**

For instance, there was an enlarged prostate case of a 62 years old man. His wife passed away when he was 56 years old, and he was diagnosed with prostate cancer at the age of 60, when his wife was not alive. During the therapy session, he admitted that during the early days of his marriage, the couple shared a fairly good relationship, but soon after they had their first child, they started facing issues in their married life. He said that his wife always complained to him for not being financially sound. He mentioned that he could not earn much through business, thus, she had to do a job to support the family. He told me that he never mentioned to her that he used to feel guilty, but he also believed that she was very demanding, and thus, it was her choice to work. He added that after starting the job, her behaviour changed tremendously. She became very rude, and they often ended up having conflicts while having their meals. Therefore, they stopped having their meals together. She had become a workaholic and thus, their married life was ruined. However, after a few years, they shared a good relationship because they didn't interact much with each other and never interfered in each other's life. Thus, he recalled that the last few years before she expired, they were on good terms and it can be said that they had a stable married life.

Root cause for his prostate disease was his subconscious anger, frustration and irritation over his wife that he continued to suppress over a period of time. He accepted that he used to miss his wife, but never told her because of his big ego. He felt rejected by his wife and suffered from a lot of resentment that led to prostate cancer.

**Healing Penile and Prostate Diseases:**

Mindfulness: Sit down in a quiet place, focus on your breath and the present moment while keeping a track of your thoughts and emotions. Remember, just like if you drink alcohol then you are causing harm to your own body, it is not going to be hazardous to the other person. Similarly, if you keep processing negative things about other people or continue to store rage, then it is going to affect your physical and mental health, not theirs. Don't let your ego spoil your relationship. Try to understand the other person's perspective and forgive them. Mindfulness can help you to cultivate a positive attitude and improve your self-esteem. Stop criticizing and cribbing over petty things, this can lead to urinary infections or other urine related issues as well.

Chakras which are imbalanced in case of prostate and penile issues are sacral chakra, root chakra, and the solar plexus chakra. Chakra meditation can help you to balance your chakras and connect with your inner voice and align your physical and spiritual energy. Nature walks can help you to open your heart chakra. Build self-confidence and tour self-esteem. Balance your throat chakra by communicating your positive feelings. Feel safe to communicate with your loved ones. Express your viewpoint and help them to understand your perspective. You can refer to the various ways to activate your chakras in the chakra section under the "Healing" Chapter of this book.

Emotion Management Technique is very effective in controlling anger. You can refer to this technique under the Healing section of the book. You can chant 'restless', 'anxiety', 'unsupported' or helpless' to surface the physical sensations and then follow the EMT steps as mentioned.

Meditation: To bring peace of mind and release your suppressed unhealed emotions, you can also practice meditations in the book's "Healing" Chapter. This will help you heal your subconscious mind deeply. These meditations will help you in forgiveness and healing your physical issues as well.

Yoga and exercises are very effective to release stress and help to maintain hormonal balance. It aids in a positive mindset and releases negative thoughts and emotions. Life can throw unexpected challenges in your way. It is your responsibility to cultivate resilience, to bounce back from adversity stronger than before. If something bad has happened in your life, it does not mean that your whole life is bad. It's just a chapter of a book, it's just a phase it will also pass.

Journaling: If you feel lonely, then start journaling your thoughts. It is an effective way to keep a track of your progress on your personal development. When you write down your thoughts and feelings, you reduce the likelihood of your unpleasant emotions being suppressed in your subconscious mind.

Transpersonal Regression therapies and counselling are the most effective ways of releasing negative emotions from your subconscious mind. Psychological therapies bring peace to your mind and help you to recover faster.

# Chapter 14
# URINARY BLADDER

## URINARY TRACT INFECTION (UTI):
## "Life is a big back to back struggle."

**Do you find yourself always complaining about your life?**

If you are suffering from urine related issues like burning sensations, less urination or frequent urination, then the root cause is your habit of cribbing about everything or everyone around you in an angry way. When you feel irritated over petty things and make a fuss about everything, most of the time, then you may suffer from urinary infections. Urinary infection could be experienced by both men and women. Common symptoms are pain while passing urine, blood, urgent urge and frequent urination. The study found that the emotions pertaining to urinary issues in both men and women were suppressed frustration and resentment towards their spouse.

**Healing:**

To avoid urinary infection, it is important for you to keep a track of your thoughts and emotions. You have to stop complaining. Well, it is easy to say and difficult to do, but it is essential for you to practice mindfulness. Avoid moaning, avoid getting stuck in a loop of negative thoughts. Change the way you respond to situations. Try it!

If you encounter any negative situation or negative person, instead of dwelling into criticism, dive into a deep introspection. Try to understand the situation or the person. Keep reviewing the incident that affected you. View it with the perspective of the other person. This will help you to understand their sentiments. It will also improve your health and capacity to think rationally.

Drinking a lot of water and increasing your fluid intake is a way of releasing all the toxins from your physical body. Ultimately, what is most important is to get rid of the toxicity in your mind.

Your solar plexus chakra, sacral chakra and root chakras are imbalanced if you are suffering from urinary problems. You have to change your plagued mindset and think positive. Avoid guilt and self-criticism. It is important to control your emotions and think positively, else it could lead to financial instability and increased relationship conflicts. Refer to the chakra section in this book to heal and activate your chakras.

## BED WETTING:
## "I need attention."

**Are you very scared of your parents, especially father?**

People who experienced issues of bedwetting displayed extreme fear of their parents; they had deep entrenched feelings of loneliness and felt like a victim. Subconsciously, there was a sense of lack of love and as a result, they are mostly attention seekers. It was observed that the clients who were bedwetting, frequently became ill as they needed attention from their loved ones. They were regarded as sentimental and dependent on others.

**Case Study**

Reva who was 8 years old, had bedwetting problems. She had tried all kinds of medications, allopathy, homeopathy, and ayurveda, but nothing could cure her bedwetting problem. As a result, she desired to undergo Regression Treatment in order to resolve the issue on a mental level. During the therapy session, an unbelievable and jaw-dropping revelation came to light that will leave you speechless.

During the treatment session, she regressed to her age of 2 months, to a time when parents were having a terrible conflict, and the poor child was terrified by the loud voices of her parents. Her mother held her very tightly and took her out of the house saying that she would divorce her father. They had recently moved to New York City, and thus, her mother didn't know anyone there, so she checked into a hotel that night. Reva became extremely sick at that time. Her mother didn't know what to do in a foreign nation and didn't have any financial assistance, so she returned home and sorted out the issues with her husband. Reva was overjoyed to be home. It's surprising but it's true that Reva, who was just 2 months old at the time, concluded that if she became unwell, then her parents would never separate. As a result, whenever her parents fought, she became ill. Her parents offered her with the best doctors and medications which cured her. Thus, she was subconsciously, scared of losing her parents and as a result she started bedwetting, for which her parents were unable to find treatment.

Reva, who was 8 years old at the time, was not even aware that she was suffering as a result of the negative inferences she had stored in her subconscious mind. It was an extremely overwhelming and shocking revelation for the 8 years old Reva. The 2 months old inner child was healed and new beliefs were formed. After a few weeks, her mother testified that her bedwetting issue was completely cured.

Through other case studies it was evident that bed wetting was experienced by individuals who were extremely scared of their parents and were attention seekers. However, there are different emotions associated with different types of urinary problems. For example, people suffering from diabetes have an intense urge to pass urine immediately. They are not able to hold it for long. As you read further, you will be able to understand the root cause of diabetes in the next chapter.

# *Chapter 15*
# DIABETES

***"I feel rejected and abandoned by my loved ones."***

**Do you wonder that you always loved your loved ones but still they rejected and abandoned you? Do you know, most of the people who are not consuming sugar in their daily life, still suffer from high diabetes?**

It is not because their pancreas is malfunctioning. The primary root cause of their increased glucose levels in their blood, is the immense bitterness that had arisen in their minds as an impact of your relationship disputes.

When you are going through turmoil in relationships with your loved ones, then automatically, your liver begins to secrete extra bile juice. Bile juice is acidic, it is only secreted in sufficient quantities to break down the nutrients of the food to help in digestion. But if bile juice is secreted in excess, then it affects the insulin and the glucose levels, which results in metabolic disturbances. Consequently, increasing high risk of diabetes.

Although you may not be consuming direct sugar but the food, vegetables and fruits you consume do contain some glucose. Even a small amount of sugar might put you on the verge of developing diabetes.

The primary root cause of diabetes is the clogging of your mind with negative emotions and thoughts which makes your life acidic. For instance, there was a case suffering from very high diabetes. Although she was taking insulin injections, her sugar level was going very high. She wished to seek a treatment to heal the root cause of her problem. So, the Hypnotherapy session was conducted.

**Case Study**

Through the session it was revealed that during her childhood she felt very lonely and abandoned by her parents. She felt that her grandparents also loved her sibling more than her and thus, developed subconscious jealousy towards him. Ironically, consciously she felt that her brother had issues with her. She mentioned after the session that she adored and cared for her brother, but he was often unkind to her. Despite her love for her brother, his frigid demeanour caused a number of misunderstandings between them. She gradually stopped seeing him and his family.

Further, in her second session, it emerged that her in-laws rejected her after she married. Her husband was likewise unsupportive. She stated that she was very kind-hearted and hence readily forgave everyone. She claimed that she continued to impress everyone in her in-laws' family, including her husband, yet they were reluctant to reciprocate. She consciously thought she was humble and forgiving, but her subconscious was filled with hate and scorn towards everyone. The root cause of her diabetes was the bitterness she was carrying in her system.

It is vital for you to be aware of your thoughts and emotions. The emotional baggage and the animosity that you are storing in your heart can put you at the verge of high diabetes.

Diabetes can lead to both weight gain as well as loss of weight. As you read further you will learn how a negative emotional mindset can affect your body structure.

**How may diabetes be avoided or healed?**

Mindfulness, self-realization and positive mindset are the key factors that can help you to avoid diabetes and if you are already suffering from high diabetes then these can help you to control your sugar levels in your blood. Awareness and acknowledgement are essential to forgive anyone. You have to overview the whole episode as a spectator or the third party. This will help you to stay neutral and understand the perspective of the other person as well. Still if you are unable to think positive then you should seek counselling or Regression Therapy.

**Psychological counselling:** Psychological counselling is a tool that helps you to vent out your emotional baggage. It makes you feel lighter and may provide you logical reasons to forgive everyone who wounded your heart. But if you feel that you have a very stern mind set and counselling cannot convince you, then you should opt for Transpersonal Regression Therapies only.

**Hypnotherapy and Transpersonal Regression therapies:** These therapies are the most effective healing techniques because they work on your subconscious mind and thus help in faster recovery. They involve inner child work and deep healing methods. They assist you in proper closures and heal your past; consequently, restoring your health.

**Diet:** Healthy diet plan and regular monitoring the nutrients you consume per day is beneficial. Remember to eat *guilt free*. Cheating meals once a week is allowed. Don't deprive yourself from eating your favourite dishes. Just keep a track of your nutrients and proportion.

**Emotion Management Technique:** Emotion Management Technique is very effective in controlling your emotions. You can refer to this technique under the healing section of the book. You can chant ‘restless’, ‘anxiety’, ‘unsupported’, ‘helpless' or 'sad’ to surface the physical sensations and then follow the EMT steps as mentioned.

**Meditation:** To bring peace of mind and release your suppressed unhealed emotions, you can also practice meditations in the book's "Healing" Chapter. These meditations will help you in forgiveness and healing your diabetes as well.

Nature walks, yoga and good sleep help to release stress and add to your healthy lifestyle. Make meditation a daily habit and balance your chakras.

Read positive and empowering quotes. Keep journaling your sentiments. It helps keep a track of your thought process.

Chakra healing and balancing will help you to clean your energies and bring calmness. You can refer to the various ways to activate your chakras in the chakra section under the "Healing" Chapter of this book.

# *Chapter 16*
# WEIGHT GAIN

***"No matter how hard I try, I never lose weight."***

**Do you wonder why, even if you treat yourself once in a while with your favourite high calorie meal and try to control your diet the rest of the time, you still gain weight?**

You are gaining weight because of stress and not because of your eating habits. Stress leads to negative emotions like frustrations and irritation which affects your glucose levels in your blood as discussed in the diabetes chapter. Moreover, stress increases secretion of certain hormones like cortisol and adrenaline which lead to fatigue and excessive weight gain. Being overweight, you feel very tired and lazy throughout the day. Consciously, you want to control your weight, but you don't feel like exercising or changing your mundane daily routines because of fatigue or body pains. You keep pacing back and forth trying very hard to lose weight but all in vain. You get up in the morning and try to stick to a diet plan, but as the evening approaches, you resort to snack cravings or unhealthy eating patterns. This occurs because the more you strive to control your mind, the more you tend to focus on your inadequacies. You keep telling yourself statements like:

*"I am going out of shape."*

*"I should control my diet."*

*"I will not look nice."*

*"What have I done to myself."*

*"I am not able to fit into my dresses."*

As a result of these negative thoughts and statements that are constantly bogging your mind, you unconsciously feel dejected and emptiness deep within. Consequently, you unconsciously fill your voids by indulging in your favourite food. Psychologically, you are actually cheering yourself up after so much unconscious self-criticism throughout the day.

**Have you ever noticed when you feel very sad, you have a craving for sweets and desserts or high calorie food items?**

When you are feeling a lot of remorse, rage or resentment due to your environment then you tend to compensate for all the bitterness by eating sweets. As you are feeling unhappy, you unconsciously try to cheer yourself up by a sweet treat or your favourite dish, which you had been avoiding due to weight issues.

**Have you ever noticed that bulge or fat is more visible in certain places of your body only, not your whole body proportionally? Do you know why you don't gain weight proportionally across your entire body?**

This is because your body will accumulate more fat only in the parts of your body where there is a void. When you are feeling an emotional emptiness in your body then different parts of your body display fat or bulge depending upon the lack, you are perceiving.

**Fat over Face, Neck and Shoulders:**

These parts of your body gain weight when there is loss of happiness. A part of you is shattered and unable to deal with it. It is also called **Crying Syndrome**. You are suppressing your voice, your soul is crying. There is a communication issue. You feel that there is no one to listen to you or you cannot share your problems with other people because they would not understand. When your smile disappears and to fill in this void by overeating or treating yourself with sweets, deserts or ice creams. Thus, the fat accumulates more on your face, neck or shoulders.

**Swollen Shoulder, Bulging Back:**

Gaining weight around your shoulders and upper back area implies you are taking on a lot of burdens of tasks on a daily basis. You are overburdened not only physically, but emotionally as well. You are trying very hard to match up to the demands of your loved ones and ignoring yourself. You are loving and compassionate, and thus, want to rescue everyone, but at the same time you feel helpless and tired of the rollercoaster that keeps you on guard. This is termed as **Responsibility Syndrome**. These overburdens result in the accumulation of excess fat in your shoulder and upper back areas.

**Arms and Chest:** Bulky chest and heaviness in your arms means that you are thriving very hard to achieve unreasonable goals. It is termed as **Fight Syndrome.** It is linked to sentiments of feeling unloved and inadequacy. When you are anonymously lacking in love, you try to be extremely available to others in order to fill up your voids with love. You strive very hard to love others and expect to be loved in return. But it is all in vain. You are good to others, but you do not get the same gesture back. You try to give love, but you do not get the same love in return. This creates even more void and lack within you, which you tend to fill up with the food which you eat, and thus, fat is visible in your arms and chest area.

**Stomach and Hip:** Most of the people think that the bulging stomach could be because of C-section delivery. Have you ever thought that if delivery was the root cause of stomach bulge, then why do men display that bulge? The primary cause of the bulging stomach is fear of loss of control. As you age, you tend to lose the grasp over your children or memory. The tasks that you could do earlier, maybe you are not able to do because of your physical body limitations. This may lead to a subconscious fear, which develops in your mind. When this loss is perceived by your mind, unconsciously it makes you indulge in overeating to fill up the voids. You feel dissatisfied and guilty. It is therefore termed as **Guilt Syndrome**.

Similarly, people have a notion that fat around their hips could be hereditary. No, that's not true. Hips also get affected by the guilt syndrome. When you feel unsupported or you feel frustrated in life, as you have to do everything on your own. You feel a lack of support subconsciously, then you tend to fill up this lack by overeating. You feel discontent and loss of control over your own life. You hope that if you will stand for others, then they will support you, but that never happens. No matter how hard you try to be there for others, but when you need them, they are never available for you. Consequently, you end up feeling angry at yourself. You dwell into self-criticism, constantly sabotaging and blaming yourself for being so good and feel guilty. You feel emptiness and you tend to fill that void with food, which leads to fat accumulation over your belly and hips.

**Heavy Thighs and Calves**: Fat accumulation around the thighs and calves means that you have a tendency of running away from the problems rather than solving them. This is called **Flight Syndrome.** If you are suffering from flight syndrome, then your mind freezes during a crisis situation, and you unconsciously escape from your issues. This can also lead to disorientation or temporary loss of memory. Heavy thighs and calves also implies that you have a fear of moving ahead in life. You are always stressed and stuck in a negative mindset. You don't want to face reality and prefer to stay in your illusionary world. Staying in illusion gives you strength and keeps you motivated to continue with your life as it comes, but unfortunately, it completely disintegrates you from your true self. Thus, you begin to gain weight in your thighs or calves.

During physical labour, you tend to feel more hungry because there is energy loss and you tend to compensate by consuming more carbohydrates to provide you energy. But do you wonder, while brainstorming in your office or during exams in your childhood, there was no physical work involved, and still you indulged in overeating? This is because although there was no physical work involved in the office or during exams, there was loss of mental energy. Thus, you compensate for the loss of energy by eating more carbohydrates, which is the primary cause of your weight gain.

**Healing Weight Gain Problems:**

It is absolutely fine to cheer yourself up by feasting on your favourite meal once in a week. You just need to be mindful of what you are consuming and its quantity. Remember to eat guilt free. The major emotion that leads to excessive weight gain is the guilt that you are attaching to the food while eating. Your thoughts create your reality.

**Healing Crying Syndrome**:

Try to communicate clearly. Feel safe to listen and express your point of view. Think positive and begin to focus on positive things around you that bring a smile on your face. Be grateful for all the valuable things in your life and express your gratitude towards them. Happiness is a choice, not the result. You have to choose to be happy. Life can be both good or bad, it is the way you choose to make it. If something bad happens in your life, it doesn't mean that your whole life is bad. It's just a chapter of your life that may be painful but it's over, you have to let go of your past and move on. Balance your third eye chakra, throat chakra, and the heart chakra. As you read the chakra section of the book, you will learn how to heal and activate these chakras. Release your sadness through the Emotion Management Technique given in the healing section of this book. Chant 'Sad, sad, sad' to bring up the physical sensation and then follow the EMT steps.

**Healing Responsibility and Guilt Syndrome:**

First of all, take a deep breath. Remember, you are worthy, deserving and your loved ones love you as you are. You don't have to prove yourself to them. Take care of your loved ones, but love yourself with the same love and compassion. Practice self-love, otherwise your heart chakra, throat chakra, solar plexus chakra and sacral chakra are blocked. In order to heal yourself, you have to be open and be receptive to unconditional love. Unconditional love is harmony and balance. It is not just a feeling, it's a way of life and a state of mind. Love is grace, and it is the favour of the universe. It is like a gift. Unconditional love lifts you out of your problems, it transforms you; it restores you and sets you free from expectations. Give and accept love unconditionally. Doing tasks to the best of your capacity, with zero expectations will liberate you from fears of being judged, fear of being right or wrong, and hence, it will never lead to feelings of not good enough, guilt or helplessness.

Emotion Management Technique: Chant 'guilt' or 'helplessness' to bring up the physical sensation and then follow the EMT steps given in the Emotion Management Technique section of the book.

**Healing Fight Syndrome:**

You do not need to be on guard. You shouldn't be so defensive. The world is not as awful as you believe. True, you cannot tolerate injustice, neither with yourself nor with others, nevertheless there is a solution to every situation and it can be achieved with calmness. There is an active inner child who is feeling injustice and unfairness. All that remains is the closure of the past dreadful childhood memory or episodes, when you encountered injustice and you could not express your sentiments. Those suppressed emotions formed the inner child, who gets triggered during similar unjust situations in your present. You just have to heal that inner child. Acceptance and acknowledgement as an adult is crucial as it would assist in gaining wisdom with an adult perspective.

Regression therapies is the most effective way to heal the inner child, while you can also heal and activate your throat chakra, heart chakra and solar plexus chakra to reduce weight. You can refer to the chakra section of the book.

Do the meditation mentioned under the 'Healing' section of the book and if you feel pain in your arms then chant 'unloved, unloved, unloved' and feel the physical sensation and follow the steps in the Emotion Management Technique section of the book.

**Healing Flight Syndrome:**

Ah ha, this one is very common. In order to heal the flight syndrome, you just need to stop running from your issues. Analyse your problems and deal with them. All the chakras from your third eye chakra to your root chakra are either partially blocked or completely imbalanced in case of the flight syndrome. Stop pretending that it doesn't bother you. Whenever there is a problem, you have a tendency to go into a cocoon. So, if you want to heal the flight syndrome, then you have to break the cocoon and face the real problems in your life. Liberate yourself from the self-limiting beliefs which are blocking you from looking at the real cause of your situation. Don't change the topic when someone is trying to point out your weaknesses. It's easy to change the topic and shut out the other person's point of view, but then you will be deprived of the real guidance that was coming towards you. There is always light at the end of the tunnel, but you have to accept it.

Heal and balance your chakras through the chakra meditation and also try Emotion Management Technique. You can chant any word 'restless', 'helpless', 'anxiety' or 'fear' to surface your physical discomfort or sensations, then follow the EMT steps mentioned in the Emotion Management Chapter of the book.

# *Chapter 17*
# ALLERGIES

## SKIN ALLERGIES AND ACNE:
## "I feel stuck in my boundaries."

Skin is your outer cover that demarcates your boundaries. When you feel stuck due to inner conflicts with questions like "Why do I have to abide by all the rules? Why can't I live my life on my terms?" then you may face skin challenges. The root cause of your skin problems lies deep in your subconscious mind. When you constantly feel irritated and stuck in your current situation, you continue to suppress your anger. This anger gradually surfaces in the form of rashes, pimples, acne or boils.

Your mind is stuck with the limitations of the outer world that makes you feel frustrated and helpless as you are not able to grip control over your situation. Everyone asks you to keep hope and faith but you feel confused and more stuck as you cannot see a single ray of light. This is when you may suffer with skin related issues.

In most cases it was observed that a common reason for mental conflicts in case of skin problem was **Separation Anxiety**. Have you been separated from your loved ones or planning for separation in near future?

It was observed that the root cause of skin allergies and acne was fear of separation from their loved ones. When you have shifted to a new place away from your loved ones or scared of being separated then you may suffer from skin rashes, or acne. It also may develop if you have lost your loved one to death. Separation anxiety triggers immense fear of loneliness. This makes you feel unhappy, irritated and helpless causing skin allergies. You wish to break your boundaries and take charge of the situation but you continue to hold back your true emotions of helplessness, anger and frustrations.

**Case Study**

There was a case of Sameena who complained of acne for the past 6 months. She mentioned that she had shifted to London for a job and she missed her family a lot. This was the reason for her acne, but it was only the trigger. The trigger of your problem is in the present, but the primary root cause always lies in your past. So, the therapy session was conducted to discover and heal the source of her problem.

Through the lovely session it was revealed that when she was 9 years old, her parents decided to send her to a hostel.

**Therapy Session:**

A deep trance state was induced and session began.

*Therapist: "How did you feel when you overheard your parents saying that they want to send you to the hostel?"*

*Client: "I felt very scared. I didn't want to go to the hostel. I loved my home and mother. I could not even think of staying without her. I felt angry over my father. I mean, how could he even think of tearing us apart?"*

*Therapist: "Did they send you to the hostel?"*

*Client: "No, but I was always terrified by this thought that if I don't behave properly, they would send me to the hostel."*

*Therapist: "How long were you feeling that terror?"*

*Client: "For about 4 years, then I understood that they would not send me away from them."*

It was evident from the session that when Sameena had to leave her family for professional reasons, the memory of Sameena's 9 years old inner child triggered. Her fear, annoyance, and rage associated with that memory surfaced, causing her acne.

It was more on the face, which simply conveyed her sadness and unhappiness, as the face is the portion of your body that holds your lovely grin. Her smile was lost, and thus, acne developed all around her cheeks and chin and upper lips.

Acne on different parts of your body represents emotions that have emerged from the past. You just need to heal your emotions to get rid of the acne problems completely. The major emotions that lead to skin allergies are irritation, frustration and helplessness. The part of your body where acne or rashes develop will convey the real problem of your life which is causing you irritation, frustration or helplessness. Hence, if you are suffering from acne or any other skin allergies in different parts of your body then just refer to the chapters of those parts, you will be able to understand the deep underlying issues of your life that are causing you skin problems.

**Healing:**

**Deep Introspection:** Separation anxiety is the primary cause of skin allergies. If you have been separated from your loved ones due to relocation, you must be conscious of your emotions. Avoid negative feelings such as annoyance and impatience. Think positively. Introspection is essential. It will assist you in analysing your situation, feelings, and actual desires. Logical thinking will assist you in understanding your situation rationally. This will allow you to make a more informed decision, and your mind will accept it both consciously and subconsciously.

Avoid stress and engage yourself in some physical exercises daily. Drink lots of water and take nature walks. Focus on your learnings. Love yourself. If you are alone then that does not mean that you are lonely. It implies that God has given you time to do self-work.

Do soul searching. All the answers are within you. You just need solace to heal the dark night of your soul. Once you get clarity in your thoughts, you will witness beautiful and vibrant radiating skin.

Focus on real happiness, treat yourself with your favourite delicacies, and most importantly, stop sabotaging yourself. Avoid cribbing, it can lead to infections. Don't resist change, don't hold back the old, let it go and embrace the new. You have taken birth to learn new things. So just cheer up and go ahead with a new enthusiasm and a new you.

Meditation and chakra balancing helps to a greater extent. Depending upon which part of your body has developed skin rash or acne, you will be able to identify your chakras that are imbalanced. You can learn about different chakras and how they can be balanced, in the chakra section of this book.

**Emotion Management Technique:** Chant 'loneliness' or 'fear' or 'helpless' to feel the physical sensation and then follow the EMT steps.

If the separation is due to the death of a loved one, then you have to attain peace by understanding, there is nothing called death. It is only the physical body that perishes, not the soul. Your deceased loved one's soul is always watching over you and guiding you as your spirit guides. I am writing this information based on my own experience. I will write about this in detail in my autobiography.

**Hypnotherapy and Transpersonal Regression Therapies:** The most effective ways for a faster recovery are hypnotherapy and transpersonal regression therapies. These therapies aid in the direct healing of your subconscious mind, inner child work and self-realization. These therapies lead you to the cathartic moments which in turn liberate you from the traumatic horrific memories and suppressed emotions. Suppressed emotion of extreme fear should be dealt effectively else it can lead to hair loss or other hair related problems.

## FOOD ALLERGIES:
## "I feel irritated by my existence."

Allergies that commonly came to me for healing were allergy to eggs, lactose and gluten. A common thread among all of the patients suffering from food allergies was some form of strife with their overall existence. Majority of them displayed a pattern of repressed childhood anger, while there were a few cases who had past lifetimes in which they had suppressed resentment towards their parents. However, there were mainly issues with the mother.

**Eggs:** The clients who were allergic to eggs carried a lot of fear and passive aggression towards their mother. Their mother was extremely dominating when they were young.

**Lactose:** The clients who suffered with lactose allergies could not have any dairy products. They were all displaying unconscious fear, frustration, and resentment towards their mother that they were not consciously aware of. The regression therapy resulted in the stunning revelation of a fact that they had previously denied.

**Gluten:** Clients who were allergic to gluten shared striking similarities in their unconscious feelings of disappointment towards their mother. They also believed that their mother never supported them. She was always silent and could never protect them from their father's restrictive mindset.

**Cocoa Chocolate or Coffee Allergy:** Clients who were allergic to cocoa stated whenever they consumed coffee or cocoa in any form, they developed a white spot or patch on their face or suffered from an upset stomach.

After conducting the therapy sessions on my clients who suffered from cocoa allergy, I observed a common link which was very interesting. I saw that all of them were given chocolates as an incentive for good grades or for any of their positive gestures or behaviour during their childhood. They associated chocolate as a reward. But unfortunately, they all grew up with a repressed sense of not being good enough and discontent. They subconsciously felt unworthy, and displayed a lack of confidence and low self-esteem that developed during the teenage years. They felt unfulfilled and undeserving of being rewarded unconsciously, and because they had connected cocoa as a reward, their physical body began to react to cocoa. Thus, the negative conclusions drawn about themselves, stored in their subconscious mind were the actual root cause of their allergy to cocoa.

Healing of food allergies is possible through awareness but in all these cases there is a triggered inner child story. Thus, Hypnotherapy or Regression therapy are the best ways to treat any sort of food allergies.

## *Chapter 18*

# DREAMS AND NIGHTMARES

***"Do you wake up in the night and feel stuck; you can't move or speak?"***

**Do you wonder why, when you wake up in the middle of the night afraid, and try to reach out to the person sleeping just next to you, you are unable to touch him or shout out for help, and you become even more anxious as you realize your voice has been suppressed?**

This happens because of the Tonic Motor Inhibition. It is the inhibitory connection of your central nervous system and your spinal cord. During sleep, your brain cuts off the electrical impulses to your motor muscles. This is why you are unable to move your arms and legs during the state of a vivid dream, thereby it prevents you from thrashing or injuring yourself.

Thus, in the middle of the night you are not able to reach out to the person sleeping next to you or even able to call out for help as your brain and muscular systems are inhibited. However, this mechanism is very beneficial as it allows you to vent out all sorts of deep traumatic emotions that are stored in your subconscious mind without any risk of any injury.

However, there are physiological dreams also in which you experience physical stimuli during deep sleep which gets incorporated as the content of your dream. But since these dreams are physiological, it is always better to avoid psychological interpretations of them. Dreams occur from the creative side of your mind, which means it is a result of the right side of your brain activity. But when you try to interpret your dream, then you use the left side of your brain, which operates on logical reasoning and analysis, therefore, very often you tend to consider your dreams as irrelevant.

The following is an amazing case study which will bring chills down your spine.

**Case Study**

In one case, a 23 years old young girl named Siya, came to me with the complaint of a recurring dream which seemed to be so real. She described her dream in which she believed herself as awake. Furthermore, everything in the room was placed exactly how it had been before she fell asleep on the current day. The books on the study table appeared unorganized, the dressing table was untidily stuffed with a lot of items, and the dressing chair faced the bed rather than the mirror. She also noticed that she was dressed in the same attire that she had been wearing that day and even the bedsheet was the same. She further mentioned that in her dream, after believing that she was awake, she tried to get out of the bed, then she realized that she couldn't move her body. She got scared and felt as if she was stuck. She tried to pinch herself helplessly, to be sure that it was all real or an illusion but could not feel the physical pain. This increased her anxiety and restlessness as she started breathing heavily with fear. She felt suffocated and her anxiety kept on increasing with the thought, *I don't know, what will happen now? I am alone, there is no one to help me, I am stuck. I feel, I will die.*

However, when her anxiousness reached its peak and physical sensations such as heart palpitations began, she eventually opened her eyes and woke up. It was then that she discovered that she had been dreaming.

During her session she told me that while dreaming, the only difference that she noticed was that the room appeared grey in colour, but everything else in the vision of the room looked like a mirror reflection. She repeatedly stated, *I feel stuck and I don't know what will happen now? I feel, I will die.*

After such an intriguing interview, her Regression therapy was conducted.

**Therapy Session:**

*A deep hypnotic state was induced and exquisite therapy began.*

*Therapist: Siya could you please repeat the most charged sentence in this statement: "I don't know, what will happen now? I am alone, there is no one to help me, I am stuck. I feel, I will die."*

*Client: "I am stuck, I will die, I am stuck, I will die, I am stuck, I will die."*

*Therapist: "Any physical sensations?"*

*Client: "Yes, I am feeling heaviness in my chest, heart palpitation, current in my feet and my hands are becoming cold."*

*Therapist: "How is this making you feel?"*

*Client: "I am feeling anxious, I am feeling helpless, I am stuck. I feel, I will die, oh my God... I feel so scared, I am stuck, I am stuck, I am stuck."*

*Therapist: "Where are you stuck?"*

*Client: "I don't know, I am blank, I can't see anything, It's very dark"*

*Therapist: "Where are you, in this darkness?"*

*Client: "I am on the bed."*

*Therapist: "How old are you?"*

*Client: "I am 4 years old."*

*Therapist: "What is happening?"*

*Client: "I woke up in the night and saw the mirror, as it was right in front of my bed, I got frightened."*

*Therapist: "Why did you get frightened, what is there in the mirror?"*

*Client: "I see someone, lying down, just next to me, on the bed; when I slept, I was alone."*

*Client cried: "I don't know what will happen now, I feel so scared, there is no one to help me, I am alone. I feel if I move this person would harm or kill me, so I hid myself in the blanket. It was very dark, I could not breathe inside the blanket, but I helplessly lay still without making any noise. I felt suffocated, I felt I will die now!"*

*Therapist: "Did you die there?"*

*Client: "No, actually it was my sister who came and slept with me as her air conditioner was not working properly. But since I was unaware of her presence, I got frightened that night, in fact, next morning when I told my family about this, we all laughed at this incident. I was always consciously aware of this incident, but never knew that I was subconsciously stuck in that memory."*

*Therapist: "Okay, so now, just hold the 4 years old Siya in your arms, who was stuck in that memory, cheer her up, accept her and integrate her. When you are ready you can open your eyes."*

**Therapist's Conclusion:**

In the current life, when Siya was 4 years old, she saw herself in the mirror that night, which frightened her to see an image of another person in the room, as she used to sleep alone in her room and other family members in their own separate rooms. Her mind was convinced that it was some unknown person in the bed, moreover it was very dark, so she could not recognise the image, hence she was terrified. Her conscious mind stopped processing. However, the Subconscious defence mechanism of Fight Flight response got activated and she tried to deal with the situation in her own way, but her conscious mind froze in that moment, feeling stuck in the mirror. After the shocking revelation, it was concluded that the inner child of Siya was feeling stuck and anxious due to which the adult was suffering.

Furthermore, during the dream state when adult Siya woke up, since she was already stuck in her past memory of the mirror, she perceived everything to be real, just like a mirror reflection. Due to the Tonic Motor Inhibition, when she tried to move her body, she could not move nor could she feel any physical pain, when she continuously pinched herself in the dream. Therefore, her anxiety and helplessness kept on increasing each time when she encountered such real dreams.

However, healing the inner child who was stuck in the traumatic memory could help the adult release from the past and trigger emotions of anxiety and helplessness. After a month, Siya confirmed that her recurrent dream stopped completely and she was not scared of sleeping alone.

**Healing Recurrent Dreams and Nightmares:**

**Mindfulness:** Be mindful of your thoughts. Awareness and the acknowledgement of the moment where your mind is stuck can help you heal. Before falling asleep, think positive. Try to think about all the good things that you did the whole day and feel the happiness growing into each and every cell, each and every muscle, and each and every tissue deeply into your body.

**Meditation and Breathing Exercises:** Meditation and breathing exercises assist you in keeping your mind calm and centred at all times. Breathing exercises help to reduce anxiety also. You can refer to the healing section of the anxiety chapter to learn this in detail.

**Music:** Listen to peaceful music before sleeping. Sound waves relax your nerves and body cells, and heals you deeply. It improves your mood swings and brings a sense of calmness and tranquillity. It brings clarity of your thoughts. Music does not only heal your mind alone, it helps you to align your mind, body and soul completely.

**Hypnotherapy and Regression Therapy sessions** are the fastest ways to treat recurrent dreams and nightmare issues. These therapies reprogram your subconscious mind and empower you through wisdom and positive understanding.

# Chapter 19
# PHOBIA

Phobia means fear. It could be fear of heights, water, flying, closed spaces, darkness, animals like lizards or worms. You are so horrified by your phobia that even a thought about it would make you feel anxious.

*Do you know there is a huge difference between Fear and Phobia?*

Like Phobia, fear can be about anything that causes you anxiety or leads to physical discomfort. But fear can be handled through your logical mind, and you can overcome your fears at your level very easily. Unlike fear, phobia is deeply rooted in your physical cellular memory and defies rationality. As a result, it cannot be healed without appropriate Psychological counselling and Regression therapies.

**Do you wonder why a few mature adults start jumping when they see earthworms during monsoons or yell like children when they spot a small little lizard or a cockroach, that is the size of their finger?**

This happens because their subconscious mind has a dreadful prior memory related to that phobia. There would be a tragic story behind their phobia, which would be triggered whenever they find themselves in similar circumstances or conditions. They suddenly freeze at that moment and cannot tolerate when someone even talks about it. Even a thought about their phobia is uncomfortable for them. All the rational reasoning of their logical mind fails in that moment; the buried terrible past memory resurfaces, triggering all of the repressed emotions linked to that memory, causing them to behave erratically.

Similarly, there is no reason for feeling frightened of darkness when you are consciously aware that you are an adult, mature enough to sleep alone, sleeping in a safe place and the doors and windows of that room are locked. But still if you feel anxiety, restlessness or other physical sensations when the lights are turned off, then that means there is a past experience which is causing you discomfort. This past experience could be in your current memory, that means there could be an inner child stuck in a traumatic past episode in the current life or it could be a dreadful past life memory. Mostly, the underlying root cause of your phobia lies in your past lives.

## FEAR OF CLOSED SPACES OR CLAUSTROPHOBIA: "I feel stuck in my life, I need space."

Claustrophobia is an extreme and irrational fear of closed spaces. Majority of the clients who suffered from Claustrophobia had a subconscious need of space. They loved their own comfort zone and resisted change. They felt helpless and suffocated in relationships if they were controlled by the other people. Most of them believed in "Live and let live." The following is an amazing therapy that will leave your heart pounding.

### Case Study

Preet was suffering from a phobia of closed spaces. She felt suffocated in caves or small rooms. She could not travel through airplanes as she felt frightened and suffocated when the doors of the aircraft were closed. She desired to travel through air, so she decided to heal her phobia through Regression therapy.

Preet was regressed to a deep hypnotic state and the session was conducted.

*Therapist: "Imagine yourself in a small closed place."*

*Client started feeling restless, her breathing went deep.*

*Therapist: "Where are you?"*

*Client: "It's very dark, I can't breathe."*

*Client started choking.*

*Therapist: "How old are you?"*

*Client: "I am 7 months old, I'm stuck in a very small place; I feel as if it's the womb... yes, I can see myself as a small baby connected with tubes...Oh! Yes, it's me in the womb of my mother."*

*Therapist: "Take all the impressions and describe how are you feeling?"*

*Preet grew out of breath and began shaking her body abnormally. She started shivering and her hands and feet grew extremely cold as if she was sitting on a large brick of ice. I gave her a warm thick blanket to comfort her.*

*She begged: "It's very cold here. Oh my gosh, I am feeling so suffocated, there is no air. Please take me out, I can't breathe."*

*Breathing heavily, she cried, "Please take me out. I will die... please, please... for god's sake! Please take me out, I can't breathe."*

*I immediately started the healing process to comfort her; the 7 months old inner child who was feeling trapped, suffocated and cold in the womb of her mother was healed and self-realization was brought to the adult Preet.*

*Therapist: "How are you feeling now?"*

*Client: "I am feeling calm now. Thank you."*

*Therapist: "Any sensations in your physical body?"*

*Client: "No, I am absolutely fine now, thank you!"*

*Session was ended with a shocking revelation.*

The therapy session was very intriguing so I became curious to confirm its authenticity. It was possible because it was her current life story. I felt it was a good chance to validate her story through the mother. I took her permission to share her session with her mother and she agreed. I invited her mother to put some light on the episode that Preet saw in her session. Preet's mother was stunned. She confirmed that what her daughter had seen in her session was absolutely spot on. She told us that when she was 7 months pregnant then she was diagnosed with pneumonia. She was admitted in the ICU and her condition was critical for six hours. Doctors informed her that her water bag had shrunk, which could lead to a possibility of miscarriage. They cautioned her that her life as well as her baby's life was in danger. They told her that her baby's heartbeat had dropped and oxygen levels were also very low and thus they would be unable to save her child. She had completely given up hope. But her prayers were answered and after a few hours of agony, medical professionals were able to rescue both the baby and the mother.

After listening to the mother's side of story, it was clear that Preet felt extremely cold during the session because she regressed to the moment when her mother was suffering from pneumonia. And since the water bag had reduced in size, Preet suffered with suffocation and choking as there was no space and air to breathe. Although the child was saved and everything was fine after a few hours, the 7 months old inner child remained stuck in the terrified memory. As a result, Preet developed a phobia of closed spaces since she was born. After a month, Preet testified that she could take a flight to Dubai. She could finally travel by air. She expressed her love and gratitude through a sweet message over the phone.

## PHOBIA OF HEIGHT:
## "I am scared of losing control."

Clients who suffered from a fear of heights had a subconscious need for control because they were afraid of losing control of circumstances.

Therefore, they always made sure that they were always in control. Most of them displayed a strong need to be recognised and thus, they were perfectionists and well organised.

This is also incredible and one of the most rewarding case studies I've ever worked on. Kelin, 28 years old who did not connect with me to heal her fear of height. In fact, she wished to seek assistance in balancing her emotions. She claimed that she was very scared of being happy. She stated, "When I am at the top of the world feeling very happy, then there is a sudden whirlpool of windfall that sucks me into deep sorrow. I feel so depressed. I want to know why my happiness always results in sadness? Why can't I remain happy for a long time? I feel so helpless." The shocking disclosure made during her therapy session was unambiguous. We were completely unaware of the unexpected twist that made everything unadorned after the session.

A deep hypnotic state was induced and the therapy session was conducted.

*Therapist: "Where are you?"*

*Client: "I am feeling very dizzy. My head is spinning, I am feeling puckish."*

*Therapist: "Look around where are you?"*

*Client: "I feel, I'm sitting on a roller coaster; everything around me is turning at 360 degrees. Like a wheel turning me upside down. I feel like I'm in the air. Oh my god, I am falling down from a building."*

*After a long pause, the session continued.*

*Therapist: "See your body on the ground, did you die?"*

*Client: "Yes."*

*Therapist: "Let's go back a few moments before you fell down from that building and see it in slow motion. Take all the impressions and describe what is happening before you fall down?"*

*Client: "I can see that I am standing at the edge of the wall. I am drunk, my head is spinning and my whole body is kind of loose as if I am dancing. Yes, I am dancing."*

*Therapist: "How are you feeling?"*

*Client: "I am feeling top of the world, I am toasting my excellent promotion by throwing a big party. One that had been long awaited. I feel so proud of myself. I am feeling so... so... Happy. I am standing at the edge and making an announcement."*

*Therapist: "What happened next?"*

*The terrified client screamed aloud: "I lost my balance and I fell off the edge."*

*Therapist: "Freeze this moment of fall and let me know what are your last thoughts as you are in the air?"*

*Client: "I am shocked, I am feeling helpless. I have no control. I know, I will die now."*

*The past life was closed and Kelin was healed.*

**Therapist Conclusion:**

It was concluded after the Hypnotic session that Kelin in her past life when she was feeling at the top of the world, feeling very happy and proud of herself, she died feeling helpless and shocked. She associated happiness with helplessness and shock. A postulate was formed in her subconscious mind that whenever she would rejoice, she would end up feeling depressed and helpless. Her mind was stuck in a loop believing she should not be happy else she would get into trouble. Hence, she developed an intense fear of being happy. She lost her balance and thus, she was unable to control her emotions.

After the session, Kelin reported that she had a severe phobia of heights. She used to avoid going for treks on mountains and always preferred to stay on the ground level. She added that before applying for her current job, she made it sure that she didn't have to go beyond the first floor. She said that she used to try going to higher floors to deal with her phobia but ultimately, she felt very giddy and puckish. It was the past life memory that triggered her unhealed emotions and caused her physical symptoms associated with that event, whenever she climbed very high. After a few weeks, Kelin sent an email expressing her gratitude as she felt strong enough and had gained courage to go for a mountain trek. She shared her pictures in which she appeared happy and she also mentioned that she didn't attract any sadness after coming back from the trek.

## PHOBIA OF WATER:
## "I feel suffocated in my life."

Clients who had a phobia of water demonstrated an unconscious sense of helplessness and being trapped in their situation. The majority of them felt stifled in their relationships or money and were struggling for a breakthrough.

Sahil who was 22 years old had a phobia of water. He said that he could not even get into the shallow swimming pool. He felt extremely nervous and heart palpitating by just a thought of going into the water. He felt that he would drown and die. Consciously, he was appalled by his own water phobia. He couldn't think of any plausible explanation for his great anxiety of approaching the shallow water of the swimming pool. So, the Hypnotherapy session was conducted.

A deep hypnotic condition was achieved, and stunning therapy began.

*Therapist: "Where are you?"*

*Client: "I can see a huge green mountain, besides a beautiful blue water lake... a small Dhaba, where I am serving people. I think I'm the owner of that restaurant."*

*Therapist: "How are you feeling?"*

*Client: "I'm feeling very happy, very joyful. I'm a very cheerful person."*

*Therapist: "Go to the moment of change. When something happened that suddenly changed your life in that lifetime."*

*The Client's body started shaking.*

*Therapist: "What is happening?"*

*Client: "I feel as if an earthquake is coming. Everything is falling down. I rushed out of my restaurant to save myself but suddenly a huge wave of water struck me. The fierce water is taking me at lightning speed. I am not able to breathe. All the mud has entered my nose and eyes. I can barely see anything now. I feel so frightened. I am worried what will happen to my family, if I die?"*

*Therapist: "Did you die?"*

*Client: "Yes"*

*The past life was closed and Sahil was healed.*

*Therapist: "Do you feel any physical sensations now?"*

*Client: "No, I am fine."*

*The session ended.*

**Therapist Conclusion:**

It was evident through the trance session that in the past life, Sahil drowned to death in the flood. He lost his control and felt helpless. He was worried for his loved ones. Thus, in his current life whenever he went near the water, his past life traumatic memory triggered and he felt scared and helpless. A few weeks after the healing therapy session, Sahil told me that he went to Goa for a holiday and he could swim in the shallow water.

**Healing phobias**

Postulates or beliefs formed as a result of traumatic past event are retained in your subconscious mind. Thus, when you encounter a similar situation in your current life, in which that notion tends to prove itself correct, then the fear gets intensified and the strong belief linked to the past traumatic episode becomes very strongly activated in your subconscious mind; as a result, you develop strong phobias based on that belief. A recurring pattern of intense emotions is experienced, once the past beliefs are triggered. Gradually, it becomes an unavoidable evil part of your life story.

You have to break the loop and change your belief system in order to break the pattern. Seeking psychotherapies or counselling does not result in the intended outcomes of entirely treating the phobias. Thus, Regression therapies are the best to heal your subconscious mind and change your negative conclusions or beliefs that are affecting your current life. This helps you to heal not only your past, but also your current life situations and brings immense sense of freedom and joy.

# Chapter 20
# SPIRITUAL GUIDANCE AND HEALING - HEALTH, RELATIONSHIPS AND FINANCIAL CONDITIONS

To break the chain of repeated misunderstandings, breakup or relationship disputes, financial losses and health problems, Transpersonal Regression therapy is the fastest technique. However, Counsclling and Psychotherapies can be considered but they are not much effective in many cases as they work through your conscious mind and thus, bring only temporary relief to your problem; moreover, they don't involve deep self-realization and inner child work, so the supressed unhealed emotions are not properly dealt.

Your mind is very powerful, you cannot fool it. Trance personal regression therapies heal your subconscious mind and thus help you to find the deeply rooted causes of the struggles in your life which are acceptable by your logical mind; hence, they bring greater clarity and awareness of the real cause of your problem and provides instant solutions.

**How to heal your Relationships?**

You cannot change your environment or other people around you but you can heal yourself to bring peace of mind; when you make changes inwards, you will notice remarkable changes in your outer world to a greater extent. When you heal yourself, then you will observe that your relationships will begin to improve. When you start understanding people's perspectives, then people around you also start understanding you. Remember your perceptions about other people is only a reflection of your own subconscious mind. It is a bitter a truth. When you heal your subconscious mind, you will see improvements not only in your relationships but also in your financial situations. You will be able to attract loving relationships as well as financial abundance and your health will also improve because every aspect of your life is connected to you. When you change then you notice changes in your surroundings.

**How to bring financial abundance?**

When you are struggling with financial issues, then the major reason is your subconscious mind stuck with unwavering emotions towards your father. To heal your financial issues, you need to liberate yourself from those repressed unhealed emotions associated with him. Father is a symbol of abundance. He is the provider who brings joy and comfort in your life. Majority of my clients who suffered with financial instabilities shared great bonds with their father in their present scenario and thus, denied having any issues with him, but after their therapy sessions it was significantly, revealed that they had past suppressed resentments towards their father. In your past if you had formed any negative beliefs linked to him or repressed unhealed emotions like fear, guilt or anger linked to him, then they obstruct your financial growth. You may be consciously aware of your issues with your father, but if you are not aware then Transpersonal Regression therapy is the beat way to discover and release your deeply rooted staunching emotions. When you heal yourself, then you will notice profound improvements in your financial conditions as well.

Most of the cases who suffered with financial instabilities had an ancestral pattern in their family lineage as a result of which even their father, mother or both parents could not enjoy their parents wealth or suffered with similar recurring financial debts. In such cases there could be oaths, curses or subconscious blockages, thus ancestral healing sessions can be done to break such patterns. These sessions have been very effective and can bring amazing results in your financial growth.

Moreover, breaking the pattern can save your children from facing similar financial sufferings later in their life.

Further, laws of attraction and manifestation can also lead to financial instabilities; your mind is very powerful..

Your mind is very powerful; it can be both creative as well as destructive. It is your choice to operate with a mindset of abundance or remain stuck in the state of lack. Universal law of attraction works on the notion of what you will focus on, will increase. It is based on the concept of vibrations. Whatever vibration you are carrying will be perceived by your surroundings and you tend to attract according. Thus, positive thinking is important. Don't focus on your lacks, instead focus on your positive reality, then you will notice that what you already have is just enough of that you need. Enough love, respect, money and bliss.

Life is a journey, it is a path of learnings and experience. You can choose to walk on your path and create beautiful memories with peace or you can remain STUCK in your negative thought patterns and perceptions, blaming yourself, other people and your circumstances. Running from your situations or blocking the people with whom you have misunderstandings is not a solution to your problem nor it is a way of moving ahead in life peacefully. Remember, you cannot fool your mind. Your mind never forgets anything, it keeps replaying the past memories and draws more negative conclusions about your surroundings. Even while you are asleep, your mind continues to process your past memories, and this is one of the reasons why when you wake up, you feel heaviness in your body.

Stern mindset and your self-created belief system will only ruin your physical and emotional health leading to a repeated pattern of loneliness, sorrow and resentment causing more misunderstandings with the other people around you. Therefore, you have to break the chain of your limited beliefs and perceptions in your mind and replace them with positive understanding. When you will understand other people, they will understand you. You are the creator of your own peace of mind, love and respect.

## LEARN TO CONTROL EMOTIONS

When you are stuck in repeated patterns of relationship disputes, health or financial issues then just feel the common emotion that is triggering in all the areas of your life and do the following Emotion Management technique. This is a highly effective technique for treating both your physical discomforts and your deeply suppressed emotions. This is an amazing approach that can help you heal your body pains as well as your mental distress.

### Emotion Management Technique:

Focus on your physical discomfort. Check, is it heaviness, pain or numbness? If you do not have any physical sensation, then simply focus on the most dominant emotion that you constantly feel most of the time. Is it fear, helplessness, loneliness, anxiety, guilt, sadness or anger? Chant that one word loudly and feel the physical sensation.

Rate the discomfort or the physical sensation on the scale of 0 to 10, where 10 being the highest and 0 being no discomfort.

Now make circles on your left- hand palm in this clockwise direction using the 2 fingers after the thumb of your right hand and say the following lines, 3 times.

**"Even though I'm feeling (pain/discomfort), because I'm feeling (emotion), I choose to heal and integrate that part of me. I love and accept myself as I am."**

Then place both hands on your stomach or heart. Close your eyes and breathe in all the positive energies through your nose, hold your breath and release the pain through your mouth. Repeat breathing in and out for 7 times.

After 7 times breathing in and out. Check your discomfort again on the scale of 0 to 10 again. Feel by how much your discomfort has reduced and give it a number.

Again, on your left hand palm through your right hand 2 fingers after the thumb, make continuous circles in the clockwise direction and say the following lines.

**"Even though I'm feeling (pain/discomfort), because I'm feeling (emotion), which has reduced a lot, but I still choose to heal and integrate that part of me. I love and accept myself as I am."**

Continue, till your discomfort comes down to 0.

## CHAKRAS

Whenever you encounter repeated patterns of mental conflicts, misunderstandings or conflicts in your relationships or financial instabilities then you tend to delve into negative thought patterns and unwavering emotions that affect your entire energy system of your existence. This energy centres are called Chakras. There are seven major chakras in your body, namely, Root chakra, Sacral chakra, Solar Plexus chakra, Heart chakra, Throat chakra, Third Eye chakra and the Crown chakra. In Sanskrit 'chakra' means wheels. These are our prime energy centres, which control the inflow and release of your energies. They are placed where your major endocrine glands are located in your physical body that secrete important hormones.

Each of these energy centres correspond to a specific frequency and colour. The front of your body accepts energy from the environment, while the back of your body releases energy. If the inflow and outflow are out of balance, it might cause a partial or complete blockage of your chakra. As a result, unbalanced chakras can create an array of physical, emotional, and spiritual issues. It is one of the major causes that may make you feel trapped in a repeated cycle of financial constraints, relationship disputes and various health problems. Thus, it is essential to heal and balance your chakras frequently.

## ROOT CHAKRA / MULADHARA:

**Keywords** – Financial issues and insecurities

This chakra is connected to your survival needs on Earth. It is placed at the base of your Spine. It takes its energy from mother Earth.

When there is uncertainty in life or fear of survival due to sudden changes in foundation, financial losses or relationship issues, the root chakra becomes imbalanced. You are insecure, despondent, agitated, and tense about the future, then your life is not steady. You appear to leap all over the place, yet nothing appears to be working in your favour. Staying in the past causes future anxiety, financial insecurity, sadness, or suicidal thoughts. As a result, when you are emotionally depressed, you may experience physical ailments such as discomfort or weakness in your lower body from hip to legs, ankles, toes, calf, knees, thighs, tail bone, anal and urinary infections.

When you feel stuck, simply begin moving in the direction of the flow. I know it's easier said than done, but your soul path is the one you least expect to travel. Life forces you to take the unknown route. Initially, it is uncomfortable to move on the unknown path, but it is better than being STUCK.

When your energies are stuck, you will feel stuck in every aspect of your life, including finances, relationships, and health. However, when you shift your direction and bring movement to your energies, you will notice a difference in all aspects of your life. When you begin to flow with a positive thinking and faith, you will experience abundance, success, peace, satisfaction, and joy in all aspects of your life.

Avoid focusing on your shortcomings because what you focus on increases. When you shift your concentration from inadequacy to all the positive things you possess in your present then you will logically have reasons to feel happy and satisfied.

Let go of your past and stay in the present. Forgive yourself and others. Forgiveness releases you from awful memories. Thank all of your karmic teachers whose cruel deeds transformed you into an emotionally powerful person. Consider how much confidence and courage you have gained in the present as a result of them. Thank them for assisting you in growing and discovering the most authentic sides of yourself.

**To balance this chakra you can do Affirmations:**

*"I enjoy every moment of my physical existence."*

*"I accept the changes in life easily."*

*"I am open and receptive to the flow of life."*

*"I feel grounded."*

*"I have faith in the Divine."*

Root chakra's colour is red, so to activate this chakra you can wear red stones in the form of bracelets, pendants and rings, like red jasper, red garnet, ruby, etc.

*Warning: Ask your astrologer before wearing these stones as it should be in accordance with your birth chart. If these stones are not advisable, then you can place the stone in the middle of your both palms and meditate.*

## SACRAL CHAKRA / SVADHISTHANA:

**Key word** – Pleasure, emotions

It represents that vibration of the prana force which aligns our consciousness to the feeling of joy for all worldly pleasures. Basically, it is the source of your emotional energy. It is the seat of your sentiments like guilt, sadness, sexual frustrations, addictions, habits. Its position is your genitals - sex organs. If this chakra is blocked, then the most probable physical issues that can be encountered could be reproductive issues, uterus related problems, pregnancy related issues, pain in lower abdomen, menstrual or menopausal issues in females or prostate and penile problems in men.

Keep your thoughts under control since they cause emotions, which cause physiological sensations. Avoid self-sabotage by developing addictions or undesirable behaviours. If something horrible happens, it does not imply that your entire life is doomed. It was just a period that was bound to happen, and so it did.

If you continue to talk about it or keep replaying the hurtful memories, then your chakras get imbalanced, which affects your entire energy system. Release yourself from your awful past memories and try to focus on positive things in your life, which bring happiness to you.

This chakra takes its energy from water. So, to activate this chakra drink lots of water or liquid intake is essential. Drink water with good thoughts. Remember water molecules change with the vibrations of your thought process. The colour of this chakra is orange so you can wear orange clothes and gemstones in any form, raw or polished. Stones like carnelian, citrine, orange obsidian, orange calcite, tiger eye, etc.

The Affirmations that can help to activate this chakra are:

*"I flow through all my sensuous experience."*

*"I accept appropriate sexual energies."*

*"I feel happy in life."*

*"I have faith in the Divine."*

**SOLAR PLEXUS CHAKRA / MANIPURA:**

**Keyword** – Control

It represents that vibration of the pranik force which aligns our consciousness to the feeling of knowing our position in life. Its position is your abdominal area above the naval, stomach, kidneys, liver, pancreas, intestines.

This chakra serves as a source of your mental energy. So, it is the repository of your past memories and thoughts. Therefore, if you continue to think negatively, it can elicit deep-seated feelings such as wrath, stress, and fear of losing control. It may impair your creativity, will power to live, and limit excitement in your life. If this chakra is out of balance, you may experience constipation, acidity, loose movements, diabetes, fatty liver, lower back problems, and other symptoms.

To activate and balance this Chakra, you must master your mind process. Think positively, concentrate on your strengths, and develop your creative abilities. Set daily goals and strive to meet them. Improve your will power. Motivate yourself. Stay in the present moment and avoid worrying about the past. Concentrate solely on the excellent things you have. Don't remain idle. Suspended activity can be hazardous, so engage in some sort of healthful activities.

This takes its energy from the Sun – Fire, you can activate this chakra by spending time in the sun. The colour of this chakra yellow, so you can wear yellow clothes and yellow stones like yellow sapphire, yellow aventurine, yellow jade, etc. in the form of jewellery or meditate on them.

**Affirmation:**

*"I take charge of my life."*

*"All is well."*

*"I feel safe to give mine and take other/s control."*

*"I have faith in the Divine."*

## HEART CHAKRA / ANAHATA:

**Key word** – Love

This chakra is the source of unconditional love and acceptance.

It is located in the heart, lungs, breast, and middle back. This chakra becomes blocked when you have emotional and trust issues as a result of relationship conflicts and misunderstandings. When you either harbour a lot of bitterness, grudges, and hatred towards the people around you, or when you are overly nurturing and disregarding yourself, this chakra gets blocked. Then you may experience physiological problems such as high or low blood pressure, heart attacks, lung ailments, chest pains, upper and middle back aches, and breast problems.

The environment provides energy to this chakra. So, spend more time in nature to stimulate this chakra. Mountains and flora can fill you with unconditional love. Spend time with people who make you happy, and do everything with no expectations. Learn to appreciate yourself. Fill yourself with love first, and only then will you be able to unconditionally spread love. Self-love is not selfish, you can care for yourself and your loved ones with the same level of love and compassion. You don't have to ignore yourself in order to love others. Accept yourself just as you are.

This chakra's colour is green. To activate this chakra you can wear green clothes or stones like green jade, green aventurine, etc.

**Affirmation:**

*"I flow in love."*

*"All is well."*

*"I accept and give unconditional love."*

*"I love and accept myself."*

*"I have faith in the Divine."*

## THROAT CHAKRA / VISHUDDHA:

**Key word** – Communication, self-esteem, confidence

It is the chakra of self-worth and self-expression. The position of this chakra is your throat and neck area. This chakra gets blocked when you are feeling dominated by authoritative figures in your life. If you suppress your emotions, feel helpless then throat chakra gets either partially, blocked or completely blocked. It could also imply excessive speaking and not listening or visa-versa, in confidence, dependent on others. If this chakra is imbalanced then the probable physical issues could be choking or dryness in throat. Pains or stiffness in shoulder, upper back and neck, diseases like thyroid, goitre, spondylitis.

It is critical that you communicate your feelings in order to balance the throat chakra. Feel free to express yourself clearly. Be flexible and open to other people's points of view while also attempting to communicate your own. Believe in yourself, you are worthy and deserved; elevate your confidence. Above all, respect yourself. You deserve to value and prioritise yourself.

This chakra takes its energy from air. You can do breathing exercises and yoga to activate this chakra. It is blue in colour. So, you can wear blue clothes and crystals or stones like lapis lazuli, turquoise, sodalite, blue jade, blue sapphire, etc.

**Affirmations:**

*"I believe in myself."*

*"I express myself adequately."*

*"I feel safe to express myself."*

*"I feel safe to listen to other's viewpoints."*

*"I love and accept myself."*

*"I'm fine, I'm okay."*

**THIRD EYE CHAKRA / AJNA:**

**Keyword** – Insight / Wisdom

It is related to Intuition, visionaries, implementers.

Its position is the centre of your forehead. When you are confused, directionless, have ideas but are unable to implement them, fear, abusive, or filthy language, this chakra might become partially or entirely blocked. It can also be closed if you do not wish to change your viewpoint. If you believe there is no point in saying anything because nothing will ever change. A stringent mental process can have an impact on your third eye chakra. If this chakra is out of balance, you may experience headaches, eye, ear, nose, tongue, and mouth problems, hair loss, excessive sweating, and pimples.

It takes its energy from knowledge giving sources like teachers, gurus, social media. So, to activate this chakra you should be open to guidance. Guidance can come in any form. You just have to accept and acknowledge it. Feel safe to change your point of view. Listening more and speaking less is the best mantra to activate your third eye chakra. The colour of this chakra is indigo. So, you can wear violet clothes and stones like amethyst, labradorite, azurite, purple fluorite, etc. to increase your intuition.

**Affirmations:**

*"I feel safe to see clearly."*

*"I feel safe to listen to others."*

*"I am open to universal wisdom."*

*"I have faith in the Divine."*

**CROWN CHAKRA / SAHASRARA:**

**Key word** – Oneness

Crown chakra relates to the feeling of oneness with the universe. The position of this chakra is the top of your head area. It takes its energy from the universe. When you have a lot of inner turmoil or lose faith in the divine process, this chakra becomes blocked, and you start having trust issues and misunderstandings with the people around you. As a result, you isolate yourself, feel victimised, lonely, and depressed. When the crown chakra is out of balance, it can cause acute anxiety, insomnia, phobias, and illusions. Common physical difficulties that may arise include brain disorders or diseases, scalp problems, hair loss, and skin problems.

The key to activating this chakra is faith. You must have faith in yourself and in the divine timing. You must take command of your life and develop your will power. Avoid sitting alone and stop procrastinating. Create new ideas and start putting them into action, meet new positive people, and socialise. Stop pointing fingers. You are the creator of your own reality.

Watch your words and thoughts about others as they are your subconscious reflections. Seek counselling, journal your thoughts. Solace is good for deep introspection but only when you focus on the positive attributes of your life. It will bring peace of mind. Remember this chakra implies *I am*. If you feel that people don't understand you then it is you who is not understanding them. So just start affirming, *I am understanding people.* If you feel people don't trust you then that means you are lacking faith in yourself or the divine process, so just start affirming, *I am faith or I trust myself.*

**Affirmations**:

*"I am open to universal oneness."*

*"I am ready to heal and integrate myself."*

*"I am safe on Earth."*

*"I am accepting and giving unconditional universal love."*

*"I love and accept myself."*

*"I have faith in the Divine."*

The colour of crown chakra is violet. You can wear amethyst, clear quartz, selenite, white agate, moonstone, howlite stones, labradorite, lapis lazuli, to clear and balance your energies.

## GUIDANCE

The gemstones, crystals, and affirmations will only work if you take the initial step towards healing yourself. To heal yourself, you need to build a strong will. These are simply tools that will guide you through the awakening process. These will cleanse your energy and guide you in the direction of the light. You have the choice to progress towards the light or remain in the darkness.

## MEDITATIONS

### Meditation for Healing Emotional and Physical Issues:

Close your eyes.

Focus on your breath.

Imagine yourself sitting on the floor in the room of your own choice where you feel very safe and comfortable.

Imagine a shaft of white light coming down from the ceiling on top of your head.

Breathe in all the positive energies and see the white light spreading all over your body from your head to the feet.

Imagine roots coming out of your toes and going down into the mother Earth.

Feel these roots going deeper and deeper. Feel your connection with the Earth strongly. Feel yourself grounded. Pause.

Imagine yourself in front of a big tunnel… Pause.

Imagine your pain or discomfort coming out from your mouth in the form of black smoke and going down into the tunnel and releasing from the other end of the tunnel, going either up or down. Feel all the negative emotions and thoughts also releasing in the form of dark black clouds.

Imagine the colour of smoke changing from black to Grey and then white.

Imagine emerald green light coming down from your head to toes and spreading all around you.

Thank the universe to protect, heal and shield you. See a silver lining all around the edge of the ball.

See yourself smiling in the green colour ball of light… Spend some time in that moment.

Then take a deep lung filling breath and feel yourself integrated with your physical body. You can open your eyes when you are comfortable.

**Instructions:** You can read out these lines and record the meditation. Then lie down in a quiet space undisturbed for at least 25 minutes and use earphones for the best results.

You can find more meditations and healing therapy sessions on my YouTube Channel – "Healing Zone by Nitika Choudhry".

## FORGIVENESS

**Meditation For Forgiveness:**

Close your eyes.

Focus on your breath.

Go to the worst moment in your life, when you felt that someone didn't understand you. You tried so hard to explain yourself to him/her but that person didn't listen to you.

As you are overviewing this situation, now:

*Ask this person, "Why did this person not listen to you? Why didn't you understand?"*

Focus on the first thoughts that are coming to you. Take all the answers to the questions that have been bothering you.

*Now overview your life after that point to see how did that event benefit you? What positive change came to you after that incident?*

*Now, feel how did it help you to grow in your later life?*

Forgive that person, thank him/her.

Do the energy exchange and let them go.

Take deep lung filling, breathe and open your eyes, when you feel comfortable.

**Instructions:** You can read out these lines and record the meditation. Then lie down in a quiet space undisturbed for at least 25 minutes and use earphones for the best results.

You can find more meditations and healing therapy sessions on my YouTube Channel - "Healing Zone by Nitika Choudhry"

## *Summary - Long Story Short*

Don't suppress your body pains or discomforts through medication or false hopes, deal with them, they can help you to reflect your subconscious issues that are causing you repeated patterns of health problems, relationship disputes and financial constraints. Keep a track of your emotions, remember they are only trigger points, the major root cause of your problems could be buried deeply in your past. Just by understanding your body discomforts, you can identify your tormenting emotions and break the recurring struggles that they are creating in your life

You have to determine whether to continue accepting positivity and growth or to fully shut everything down and escape into your cocoon, where you feel comfortable but there is no growth, happiness, or peace of mind. It's like living in your own illusionary world which only leads to loneliness and insecurities. To achieve real peace of mind, satisfaction and joy, you have to break this illusionary wall and face reality. Reality could be challenging as it's uncertain and unknown to you but it would be an opportunity to grow and evolve.

Life is an adventure, and each phase is a new chapter. Let it unfold as it ought to be. Just release yourself from the shackles of your past and resistance. Don't hold yourself back, be open to the new opportunities and have faith that you can conquer them with your strength and confidence.

Remember you are the creator of your own reality, so think positive. It's easier said than done. Life is unpredictable and sometimes brings you to a certain point where you tend to give up on yourselves and the people around you. But thinking negative, blaming others or continually replaying past traumatic memories will only damage your health.

Liberate yourself from your painful past and maintain a healthy mindset. It will bring you peace of mind, improve your relationships and your financial conditions;

Keep smiling, stay happy and blessed, always.

# Authors Bio

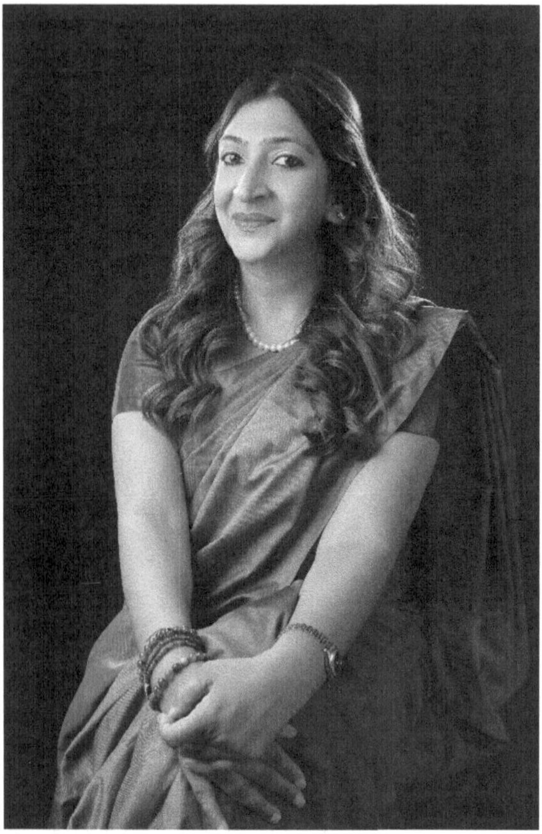

The founder of Divine School of Light, Nitika Choudhary is a certified Clinical Psychologist and Transpersonal Regression Therapist with over 21 years of dedicated experience in the field of psychology. She has done her graduation in Psychology Honours from Kamla Nehru College, New Delhi in 1998 and Masters in Clinical Psychology. She has worked in VIMHANS Vidyasagar Institute OF Mental health, Neuro & Allied Sciences Hospital in New Delhi. Her creative instincts pushed her towards few design courses along with her studies but in her heart, she wanted to contribute to the society.

Her zeal to work for people made her pursue Integrated Clinical Hypnotherapy from EKKA formally known as CHII (California Hypnosis Institute of India). She was honoured and recognised by the International Medical and Dental Hypnotherapy Association - USA TASSO Institute (Netherlands).

Nitika Choudhary is also a certified Grandmaster Reiki Healer, Advance Tarot Reader and Coach Advance Angel Card Reader and Therapist, Numerologist, Astrologer, Motivational Speaker and the founder of Divine School of Light, a healing centre and an online coaching platform that conducts Transpersonal Regression therapies, Relationship counselling ,Physical and Mental Healing sessions, Tarot Readings and Coaching, Angel Card Reading and Healings, and Numerological and Astrological Predictions. The school imparts knowledge about Self-hypnosis and other modern healing modalities to empower oneself and lead a healthy and peaceful life.

By virtue of this Divine School of Light, she wants to help people believe in energies. the school teaches about our central energy system, chakras, and aura. This school emphasizes Ancient Vedic and healing concepts to align our mind, body, and soul. This school makes people understand healing techniques in the most scientific way, to bring your logical mind and heart on the same page.

She also conducts spiritual awakening classes to bring soul awareness to the people. She has a YouTube Channel – "Healing Zone by Nitika Choudhary" in which she has been uploading free therapies and healing sessions to heal the subconscious mind. These help to increase peace of mind, happiness, exercise motivation, build confidence, and relieve stress.

After extensive research on all her clients, she observed a similar emotional pattern displayed by all of them that was causing specific physical symptoms in them. This inspired her to write this book so that it could make people aware of how their buried past can be devastating. With the help of her case studies, she has tried to help people clearly understand how their suppressed emotions and self-limiting beliefs can lead to various health issues and diseases as well relationship disputes and financial instabilities.

# Acknowledgements

**Letter Of Gratitude**

*"I would like to express my gratitude to all my lovely Teachers, Guides and My Guru Ji for guiding me at every step of my life, both professionally and personally. I am grateful to all my clients, soul family, and friends who helped me finish my research and validate my findings. Last but not least, I want to thank my twin flame from the bottom of my heart for inspiring me to write a book on my studies.*

*My twin flame is the source of my inspiration who inspired me to become an author today, and I will be publishing my next book based on my magnificent twin flame journey shortly."*

- ***Jai Guruji, Shukrana Guruji***

# Quick Look

## *Dictionary to most of the health problems and their emotional Causes:*

**Abdominal pains**- Feeling frustrated , scared and extreme anxiety.

**Accidents** – Self anger/ Guilt.

**Aches** - Guilt, need for love.

**Acne** – Irritation, separation anxiety and feeling stuck in your boundaries.

**Addictions** - Extreme fear and running from reality.

**Aids** - Sexual frustration and guilt. Not approving yourself.

**Allergies** – Irritation, anxiety and feeling stuck in your boundaries.

**Alzheimer's Disease** - Refusing to accept reality and hopelessness.

**Anaemia** - Lack of happiness, lack of desire to live, feeling that life is terrible.

**Ankle** - Not feeling supported, guilt and inflexibility.

**Anorectal Bleeding** - Stored past anger.

**Anorexia** - Loss of will power, extreme fear, feelings of rejection and self-hatred.

**Anus** - Refusal to release the past angers and resentment.

**Anxiety** - Lack of trust.

**Arms** - Feeling unloved; need to stand up for self.

**Back Problems** - General lack of support.

> **Upper** - Lack of support and helplessness; overburdened with responsibilities.

**Middle -** Guilt and feeling of stuck, fear of death.

**Lower -** Lack of financial support; helplessness and frustration.

**Bad Breath -** Angry and revengeful thoughts, using abusive language or negative words. Sarcastic and critical in nature.

**Baldness -** Extreme fear and stress.

**Bedwetting -** The fear of parents, attention seeker, loneliness.

**Bites -** Fear.

**Animals -** Self anger.

**Bugs -** Guilt.

**Blackheads -** Stored anger.

**Bladder Problems -** Anxiety, fear of loneliness and criticism.

**Bleeding -** Lack of happiness.

**Blisters -** Resistance and feeling agitated; feeling unloved.

**Blood Pressure:**

**High -** Excessive stress due to overthinking as problems never end.

**Low -** Limited beliefs and negative conclusions formed during childhood.

**Body Odour-** An extreme fear of rejection and being judged.

**Boils -** Stored anger and irritation.

**Bone Problems:**

**Fractures -** Passive aggressive behaviour; rebelling against authoritative figures.

**Osteoporosis -** Mental pressures and lack of support.

**Bowels -** Undigested thoughts.

**Brain -** Analytical mind; refusal to accept.

**Breast -** General ignorance of your needs and prioritizing others.

**Right breast -** Stress due to husband. Feeling that the husband is not giving time or you are not able to spend quality time; fear of an extramarital affair of your husband.

**Left breast -** Issues with the children. Not being able to spend time with children; feeling a lack of their love.

**Breathing Problems -** Overburdened with responsibilities; helplessness and irritation.

**Bronchitis -** Anger and irritation over loved ones.

**Bruises -** Self-anger.

**Burns -** Self-anger

**Cancer -** Deeply stored grudges, resentment and hatred.

**Car sickness -** Fear of feeling trapped.

**Cataracts -** Fear of seeing reality.

**Cholesterol -** Extreme fear and not accepting happiness in life.

**Chronic Diseases -** Refusal to change.

**Cold-** Irritation and feeling of being ignored.

**Colon -** Fear of letting go of the past.

**Coma -** Extreme fear; trying to escape when it is very painful.

**Congestion -** Irritation and stored anger; suppressing emotions.

**Conjunctivitis -** Anger over life.

**Constipation -** Trying to hold on to ideas. Replaying the past memories.

**Corns -** Stored anger and negative thoughts of your painful past.

**Cough -** Suppressing your emotions; not being able to express your ideas freely. Irritation and anger towards life.

**Cramps -** Fear and tension.

**Crying -** Stored sadness.

**Cuts -** Self-punishment.

**Cyst -** Stored past wounds and anger.

**Deafness -** Not wanting to listen to others' perspective.

**Depression -** Lack of will power and hopelessness.

**Diabetes -** Anger over the loved ones; need to control.

**Diarrhoea -** Extreme fear and feeling of loneliness.

**Dysentery -** Extreme fear and feeling of being trapped.

**Ear -** Refusal to listen to others point of view.

**Eczema -** Mental pressures and anxiety.

**Elbow -** Inflexibility in adapting to the new.

**Endometriosis -** Insecurity and disappointment; frustration and lack of creativity.

**Epilepsy -** Refusal to flow in with life. Rejection, struggle and self-anger.

**Eye -** Refusal to see reality; feeling that nothing's going to change.

**Face -** Lack of happiness; lost smile.

**Fainting-** Extreme fear; not being able to cope with the situation.

**Fat -** Stress and overthinking.

**Fatigue -** Procrastination and boredom.

**Feet -** Fear of future.

**Fever -** Stored anger.

**Fibroid, tumours -** Stored anger.

**Fingers:** Generally focusing on too much details; a need to be a perfectionist.

> **Thumb -** not feeling supported.
>
> **Index finger -** Ego, stubbornness and fear.
>
> **Middle finger -** issues with people around especially, with longest relationships.
>
> **Ring finger -** issues with spouse.
>
> **Little finger -** emotionally very sensitive.

**Fistula -** Stubbornness and Stored anger.

**Flu** - Irritation and frustration; fear of loneliness.

**Food poisoning -** Feeling anger over the loved ones and not being able to digest the ideas of life.

**Foot Problems:** Fear of future.

**Fractures -** Rebelling against authoritative figures.

**Fungus -** Refusal to change the self-limited beliefs.

**Gallstones -** Negative thoughts, stored anger, nursing old wounds.

**Gas pains -** Extreme fear and frustration.

**Gastritis -** Fear of the unknown, waiting for things to settle but uncertainty.

**Genitals -** Sexual frustration, unsatisfied, self-anger and guilt.

**Glands -** Suppressing your emotions; nothing's going to ever change.

**Goitre -** Suppressed emotions, feeling like there is no use of saying.

**Gray hair -** Extreme fear, pressures and stress.

**Gum problems -** Stored anger, not able to stand for self.

**Hands -** Multitasking, working very hard to thrive in life, ambitious to achieve certain goals.

**Headaches -** Inner conflict, always thinking about something or someone.

**Heart -** Stress, betrayals, lack of love; relationship conflicts.

**Hepatitis -** Intolerance towards domination; stored anger and helplessness.

**Hernia -** Stored old wounds, anger, relationship conflicts.

**Hip -** Feeling unsupported, fear of future; imbalanced mind state.

**Hyperthyroidism -** Communication issues and fear.

**Hypothyroidism -** Suppressed emotions, feeling like there is no use of saying.

**Impotence -** Sexual pressures, fear, guilt; social beliefs and customs.

**Infection -** Anger, irritation, feelings of not being recognised.

**Inflammation -** Fear, replaying memories of stored wounds.

**Ingrown Toenail** - Stored anger, feeling injustice.

**Injuries -** Guilt and self -punishment.

**Insomnia** - Stress, depression, anger over God, injustice, fear of future.

**Intestines -** Making important decisions, fear of future and uncertainty.

**Itching -** Irritation, separation anxiety, remorse, loneliness.

**Jaundice -** Intolerance towards parents' domination, stored anger.

**Jaw -** Stored anger and feelings of revenge.

**Joints -** Fear of change, inflexibility, stubbornness.

**Kidney -** Criticism, dissatisfaction, childish behaviour.

**Kidney Stone –** Stored anger, guilt towards parents or siblings.

**Knee -** Ego and stubbornness.

**Left Side of the Body -** Stuck inner child, imbalanced feminine energy, suffering is self-created.

**Leg -** Fear of moving ahead in life.

**Leukaemia -** Anger, limited belief system and loss of will power.

**Liver -** Dominating parents; stored anger, very revengeful tit-for-tat kind of nature.

**Lock Jaw -** Stored anger, feelings of revenge.

**Lump in Throat -** Stored resentment and hurts; not expressive.

**Lung -** Overburdened responsibilities, grief, feeling unloved.

**Malaria -** Anger and problems with nature.

**Menopause Problems -** Fear of losing femininity, nurturing too much.

**Menstrual Problems -** Rejecting femininity, anger, strong masculine energy.

**Migraine -** Half consciousness is missing; always thinking of someone else. Not staying in the present.

**Miscarriage -** Fear of future, masculine energy is high.

**Mouth Problems -** Extreme anger; eating angry words or using abusive language.

**Muscles -** Inflexibility, resistance to change.

**Nail -** Suppressing anger; fragile in nature; insensitive in nature, "Handle with care" type of person.

**Nail biting -** Nervousness, fear of parents.

**Nausea -** Extreme fear.

**Neck -** Resistance to change, rigid thought process, like a bull head.

**Nerves** - Frustrated with life process, given up, hopelessness.

**Nose Problems:** Generally feeling unrecognized.

> **Bleeds** - Feeling ignored, irritation.
>
> **Runny** - Frustration and irritation; can't take it anymore; surrendering.
>
> **Stuffy** - Irritation, holding on past grudges.

**Numbness** - Feeling blank, confused; absolutely no clarity.

**Osteoporosis** - Feeling unsupported, dependent on others.

**Ovaries** - Rejecting feminism, need of high masculine energy, issues with siblings, mother or kids.

**Overweight** - Stress and past emotional wounds.

**Pain** - Guilt, frustration and helplessness.

**Pancreas** - Stored anger due to bitterness in life.

**Paralysis** - Resistance to change, fear, escaping from present.

**Parkinson's Disease** - Fear and running from the present; loss of control.

**Piles** - Storing old hurts and wounds; just don't want to forgive; stubbornness in releasing the past.

**Pimples** - Irritation, anger.

**Pituitary gland** - Fear of loss of control and too much analytical.

**Pneumonia** - Overthinking, worries and fear.

**Prostate** - Rejection from wife, guilt, frustration and helplessness.

**Polio** - Hatred, jealousy, clogged thinking.

**Psoriasis** - Stored anger, feelings of rejection.

**Rabies** - Stored anger and violent in nature.

**Rash** - Irritation and stored anger.

**Respiratory Ailments** - Overburdened with responsibilities.

**Rheumatoid Arthritis** - Resistance to change; stubbornness, ego.

**Rickets** - Feeling unloved and insecure.

**Right Side of the Body** - Problems due to external factors, people or environment. High, masculine energy; domination.

**Root canal** - Stored anger and feelings of revenge.

**Sciatica** - Too much running mentally or physically.

**Scratches** - Irritation due to rough life.

**Sea sickness** - Extreme fear, mostly related to past life.

**Seizures** - Trying to escape from family or the present.

**Shin** - High standards of living and pride.

**Shoulders** - Overburdened with responsibilities.

**Sinus problems** - Irritation, feeling unrecognized.

**Skin** - Separation anxiety, irritation; fear of going out of your boundaries.

**Slip disc** - Feeling unsupported.

**Snoring** - Stubbornness and resistance to change. Don't want to let go of wounded past.

**Sores** - Suppressed anger and resentment.

**Spasms** - Extreme fear.

**Spinal Curvature** - Feeling unsupported and overburdened with responsibilities.

**Spine** - Inflexibility.

**Spleen** - Obsessive thoughts.

**Sprain** – Passive aggression and resistance to change.

**Sterility** - Resistance to change.

**Stiffness** - Rigid thought process.

**Stomach** - Negative thought process, stress and tension.

**Stroke** - Hopelessness, helplessness; refusal to the change.

**Sty** - Stored anger.

**Suicide** - Helplessness, hopelessness, giving up; escaping from reality.

**Swelling** - Stored anger over old hurts and past memories.

**Teeth -** Stored anger and feelings of revenge.

**Throat -** Communication issues; suppressing emotions.

**Thyroid -** Suppressing emotions as there is no use of saying anything; Feeling like nothing's going to change.

**Tics, Twitches -** Extreme fear.

**Tinnitus -** Stubbornness and refusing to listen to others.

**Toes -** Focusing on minor details.

**Tongue -** Stored anger.

**Tonsillitis -** Extreme fear and anger.

**Tuberculosis -** Need for revenge.

**Tumours -** Outburst of stored anger.

**Ulcers -** Extreme fear and stone anger; limited beliefs.

**Urinary Infections -** Cribbing and criticizing in nature.

**Urticaria -** Extreme fear of loneliness.

**Uterus -** Issues with mother siblings or children; rejecting feminism.

**Vaginitis -** Issues with the husband; sexual guilt, self-anger.

**Varicose veins -** Hatred towards life.

**Vertigo -** Feeling unsupported, fear and helplessness.

**Viral infections -** Stored anger and resistance to change.

**Vomiting -** Extreme fear.

**Weakness -** Extreme fear and helplessness.

**Whiteheads -** Secretive or hiding something.

**Wisdom tooth -** Stored anger.

**Wounds -** Guilt and self-punishment.

**Wrists -** Feeling restricted and in a few cases, it could be issues with the parents.

# Connections

**Instagram:** nitika_healing_zone_/

**Facebook:** Healing zone by Nitika

**Website:** www.divineschooloflight.com

**Youtube:** @healingzonebynitikachoudhary

**Whatsapp:** Spiritual Awakening by Nitika

chat.whatsapp.com/FK0q0ZOBI8oHeQdZ0lPO3A

**Email:** divineschooloflight@gmail.com

# NOTES

# NOTES